THE 4-WEEK GUT HEALTH PLAN

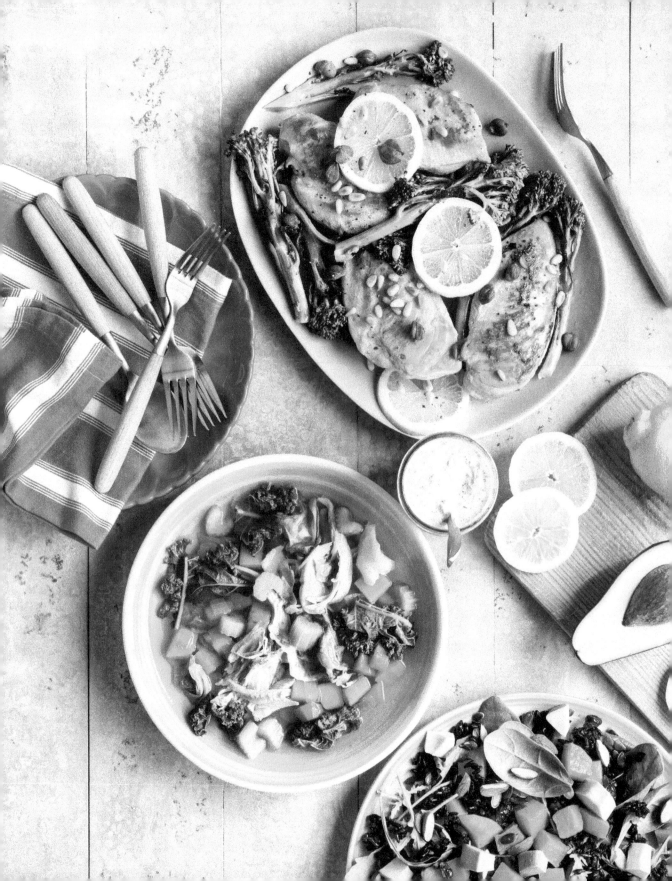

THE 4-WEEK

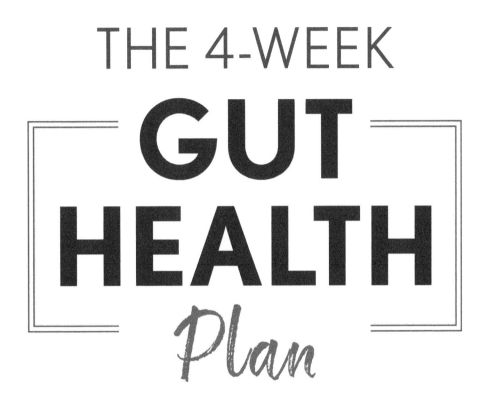

GUT HEALTH

Plan

75 Recipes to Help Restore Your Gut

Kitty Martone

PHOTOGRAPHY BY NADINE GREEFF

ROCKRIDGE PRESS

Interior and Cover Designer: Lisa Forde

Art Producer: Karen Beard

Editor: Marjorie DeWitt

Photography © 2019 Nadine Greeff. Author photo courtesy of Kat Tuohy.

ISBN: Print 978-1-64152-591-6 | eBook 978-1-64152-592-3

To my favorite person, my husband, who tested all the recipes in the book—

but more important, tested the ones that didn't make it into the book and

found kind and honest ways to say, "Nope." I love you, Charlie.

And to my father: truly, truly my biggest fan! I love you, Pops.

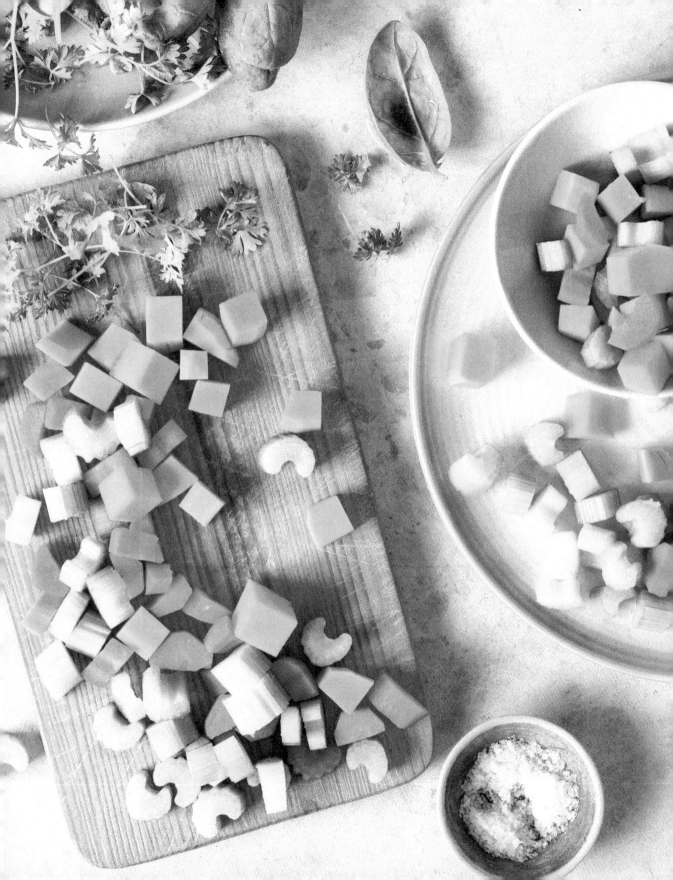

Contents

Introduction

For a few years, I worked in a center that helped rehabilitate children with various disorders and diseases. It was a humbling and eye-opening experience. The kids' ailments varied from cerebral palsy to spinal cord injury to varying degrees of autism, but a common thread among them all was gut dysbiosis. Some of the mothers of these children were nothing short of superheroes. Their seemingly tireless efforts to find any solution that might bring digestive relief to their children among much larger issues were amazing. They knew the importance of gut health, and something as simple as facilitating a bowel movement became a daily goal. It affected the children's mood, appetite, sleep, focus, and immunity—gut health *mattered*. It was a message for all of us—not only about how profoundly important gut health is to our every daily action, both conscious and subconscious, but about how hard we must work to achieve healing and harmony in our guts.

The irony was that these parents were working so hard to ease their children's suffering, all while experiencing their own digestive distress. I can only imagine what the stress they were enduring was doing to their own tummies. And isn't this the way it goes? We are all so busy with our families, jobs, and finances that we neglect our own needs. And then we reach a day when we can no longer ignore our own issues because . . . well, our issues won't let us. That's when the problem becomes a constant struggle, whether it's chronic visits to the bathroom or not being able to go to the bathroom for days on end. Maybe it's uncomfortable bloating from eating the simplest of foods or the countless other symptoms that affect our daily routines.

If this seems all too familiar, you are not alone. In fact, sadly, one recent survey by a biopharmaceutical company revealed that 74 percent of Americans live with digestive distress.

Maybe you have been given a diagnosis of a digestive disorder; even if you haven't, maybe you know something isn't right and can no longer ignore the issue. Either way, in this book, you have stumbled upon a wonderful resource to help guide you on a journey of healing. A medical doctor can certainly help get you out of crisis, and everyone with health concerns should see their medical professional for a full evaluation. However, the only way to truly resolve these

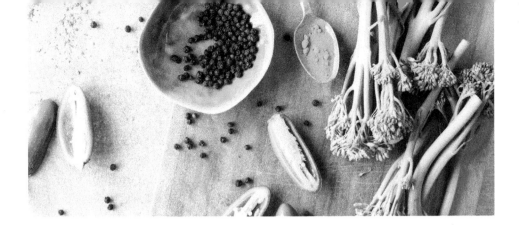

digestive disorders is to get to the root cause and begin your healing from there. Anything else would be treating the symptoms while masking the true underlying problem.

This book will give you the tools you need to begin the process of real healing. It will simplify the daunting task of planning meals and figuring out what you should and shouldn't eat. It will also solve the issue of finding recipes that work with your new lifestyle. Specifically, this book offers:

Very clear instructions for 4 weeks of meals, including shopping lists and daily menus to take the guesswork out of what to eat

Customizable meal plans that accommodate different dietary and treatment needs

Practical advice and troubleshooting tips for managing and sustaining your new diet and lifestyle through life's ups and downs

Ways to stay on top of your day-to-day routine

Tips for managing food prep for yourself and your family

Options to be smart about your food choices when prepping is not possible (e.g., grabbing food on the go or creating a contingency plan)

Ways to make the most out of vacations

Strategies for surviving social and work events and family holidays

Suffering from digestive distress or being given a diagnosis of a digestive disorder is difficult. This can be a very challenging process. It takes a great deal of effort to research, plan, and create a new lifestyle, especially when you're not feeling great. Knowing that, I wrote this book for you—to help you through this challenging phase by offering my thorough research, my tried-and-true meal plans and recipes, and my words of encouragement and guidance. You've got this!

PART

1

The Importance of Gut Health

The wonderful and vast world of your gut consists of trillions of organisms that not only help with digestion but are key players in your hormone health, nervous system, and immune system. All the organisms in your gut roughly weigh about two to three pounds, which is ironically the average weight of the human brain. All these microbes collectively act as another organ that affects every system of the body.

In this part of the book you will learn all the different ways a disturbed microbiome contributes to ailments you may suffer from and how to heal and begin to restore balance.

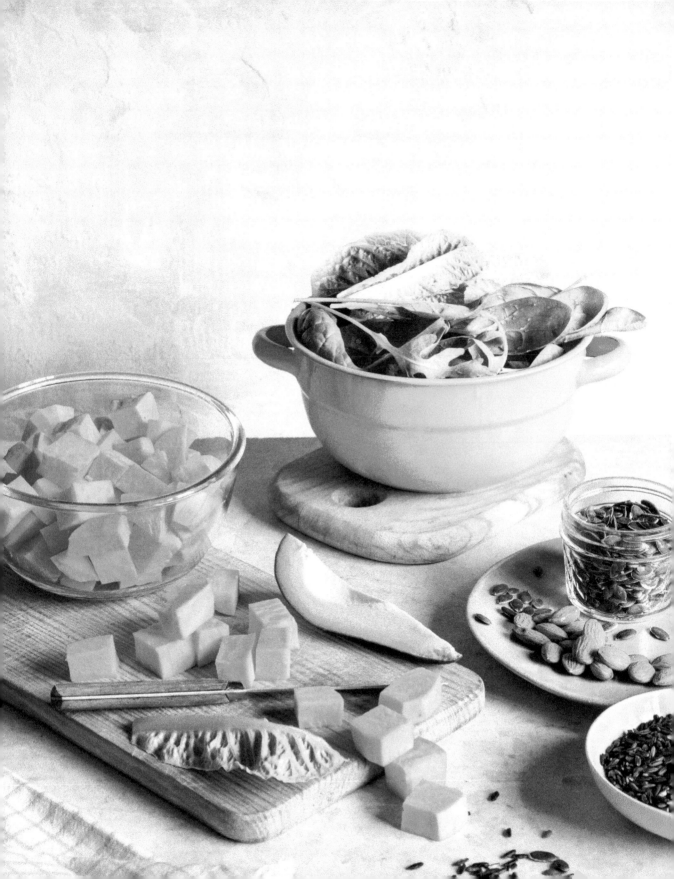

Your Gut and You

The subject of the gut can be overwhelming—and having access to incredible amounts of information at our fingertips can be daunting. The idea that there are trillions of microorganisms living on us and in us is creepy to begin with . . . but the idea that they can run amok when they aren't nourished correctly can be a bit scary! However, the most important thing to remember is that we have full control over all of it. Think of your fork as a magic wand that, when wielded properly, can bring balance to your microbiome and, thus, your health.

An Overview of Your Gut

When you hear the word "gut," you might think about the spare tire that spills over our jeans, but more properly, "gut" refers to the entire digestive tract, alimentary canal, or gastrointestinal tract—basically, from our mouth to our back door. We have about two to three pounds of microbes in this tract, good, bad, and neutral. They live in our mouth, throat, stomach, and all the way down to our rectum, though most live in our colon, also known as our large intestine.

Let's take a moment to review a little anatomy. Right after our stomach, we have our small intestine. The small intestine is about as big around as the average middle finger, but it's quite long: 20 feet long, to be exact. It is nicely folded and tucked under the stomach and lies on top of the large intestine. And while the large intestine is only 5 feet long, it's much larger in diameter. It is shaped like a horseshoe in the lower abdomen. After the large intestine comes the end of the colon and the rectum and anus. Most mineral and vitamin absorption takes place in the small intestine, while most of the liquid from the food we eat is taken up in the large intestine. Common ailments in the small intestine are celiac disease, Crohn's disease, intestinal blockage, irritable bowel syndrome (IBS), ulcers, and small intestine bacterial overgrowth (SIBO). The more common ailments in the large intestine are colon cancer, ulcerative colitis, polyps, and diverticulitis.

The Microbiome: A Colony of Friendly Bacteria

The "microbiome" is what we call all the microorganisms that live in your digestive tract. These microscopic organisms consist of about 80 percent beneficial bacteria and fungus or yeasts, and 20 percent are neutral bacteria and pathogens. The beneficial bugs are doing all sorts of great things for you, like helping digest food, making vitamins, defending you from the pathogens or "bad bugs," or helping produce hormones; others are couriers, sending messages to the brain and other bacteria to carry out various functions. They are all like factory workers, each with its own job. Even the pathogens have a specific purpose. For example, the "bad bug" *E. coli* helps us digest the dairy protein lactose. When your microbiome is healthy and functioning optimally, the "bad guys" are kept in check by your "good guys"; everyone gets along and works together properly.

But when we start to neglect our diet, use too many antibiotics, and have too much stress, the good guys can get run down, a condition called "dysbiosis." The bad guys see an opportunity and start to act out. This is when imbalance, illness, and, ultimately, disease begin to manifest. Imagine you have a beautiful well-tended garden with a nice mix of plants, happy bumblebees, and more. If you go away for a while, you may come back to a mess of weeds and pests overtaking your rosebushes. Your garden will always have insects and weeds lurking about, and they even contribute to the ecosystem in many ways—balance is important. It's when we lose that balance that the garden becomes messy, overgrown, and even dangerous. The same is true for our own bodily ecosystem. The goal isn't to kill off every pathogen, but rather to find a healthy balance.

Living with Illness

Many gut diagnoses are brand-new in modern medicine, and what used to be rare is now commonplace. Occurrences of celiac disease, SIBO, IBS, antibiotic-resistant digestive issues, ulcerative colitis, and food allergies and sensitivities are skyrocketing. Often, people leave their doctor's office with a misdiagnosis or a diagnosis of "unknown issues." This isn't the fault of the doctors; we, as a nation, have arrived at a new frontier in health. We can make educated guesses about why—having to do with declining food quality and overuse of chemicals. But these are only guesses; proper testing has never been done on all the variables we face with our food supply. Add to that our individual genetic predispositions—maybe a sensitive stomach or acid reflux runs in your family—and then add to *that* your daily exposure to stress and your personal stress history—perhaps you have PTSD or some other emotional trauma. And how many of us have taken countless courses of antibiotics? These variables can make it very difficult to determine what you may be suffering from and what to do about it.

We can all relate to feeling a little intimidated about questioning our doctors during an appointment. Just remind yourself that your doctor isn't the one who will have to live with any decision you make for you or your family's health. Write your questions down beforehand, keep them concise and specific, and be kind and respectful with your inquiries. Don't be afraid to get second opinions. Here are some ideas:

1. If you are being prescribed an antibiotic, express your concern about whether it's necessary. "Can we do a culture and sensitivity test to make sure I don't have a virus that may not respond to an antibiotic?"

2. If you do need an antibiotic, ask, "How can we be sure this antibiotic will be the correct one for the job?"

3. "What are the different tests you offer to determine various gut issues?"

4. "Prior to taking any medications, would you suggest trying dietary changes or natural remedies?"

5. "If not, what are the side effects of the medications and how quickly can I expect to stop taking them?"

Common Causes of Gut Dysfunction

It is very difficult, if not impossible, to pinpoint the exact reason a person may fall victim to a gut imbalance, disease, or disorder. Individual differences play a large part: We don't yet know what may cause one person to have gastroesophageal reflux disease (GERD) and another to have IBS. However, in general, we can say that your biggest risks for digestive issues are almost always poor diet, poor digestion, and a sluggish gut. High stress levels, antibiotics, and certain other medications may also increase your risk of developing some type of gut dysbiosis. According to Johns Hopkins University, up to 20 percent of adults worldwide reported symptoms consistent with IBS. Thankfully, we've begun to recognize the extent of the problem and find ways to deal with it—naturally!

Signs of an Ailing Gut

Some of the more common, well-known signs of an ailing gut include:

- Gas
- Bloating
- Constipation
- Diarrhea
- Cramping and abdominal pain
- Acid reflux or heartburn
- Nausea
- Discomfort when eating
- Runny, hard, and/or overly smelly stools

Some of the less well-known signs include:

- Hemorrhoids
- Food allergies
- Upper shoulder pain
- Skin imbalances, like eczema, acne, and skin eruptions
- White-coated tongue
- Bad breath
- Receding gums
- Dental infection and cavities
- Thrush or yeast infections of the mouth or anus
- Head fog or malaise
- Chronic fatigue
- Unexplained weight loss or gain
- Leaky or runny nose
- Chronic colds that turn into chest colds
- Autoimmune issues
- Hormone imbalances, like thyroid problems
- Gallstones
- Rosacea

Common Gut Illnesses

If you have chronic issues with one or more of the symptoms listed previously, you could be at risk for receiving a gut-related diagnosis. These are some of the more common gut diagnoses today:

GASTRITIS is a result of an inflamed stomach lining. It may cause bloating after meals, burping, tightness in the belly and chest, gas, or abdominal pain.

GASTROESOPHAGEAL REFLUX DISEASE (GERD) is a result of stomach acid chronically bubbling up from the stomach to inflame the esophagus. It causes chest pressure, nausea, burning in the chest and throat, foamy saliva, bad breath, burping, and sometimes headaches.

SMALL INTESTINAL BACTERIAL OVERGROWTH (SIBO) is the result when certain bacteria that should be in the large intestine make their way up to the small intestine and grow out of control there; this causes food intolerances, bloating, pain, gas, burping, and diarrhea.

SMALL INTESTINAL FUNGAL OVERGROWTH (SIFO) is a result of a fungal overgrowth like candida in the small intestine. The symptoms are similar to those of SIBO.

H. PYLORI **OVERGROWTH** is caused when bacteria that is supposed to be in our stomachs get too enthusiastic and begin to cause stomach ulcers and lesions. Ironically, this can be a result of chronic low stomach acid, or of poor diet, chronic stress, or medications. Symptoms of ulcers are severe pain in the upper abdomen, sides, or shoulders, as well as vomiting, diarrhea, and loss of appetite.

CELIAC DISEASE (ALSO KNOWN AS CELIAC SPRUE OR GLUTEN-SENSITIVE ENTEROPATHY) AND GLUTEN SENSITIVITY are autoimmune diseases that can have a genetic component and can be inherited and passed down. Celiac disease is a lifelong condition with no known cure, though it can be managed. Gluten sensitivity does not necessarily have to be inherited; it's increasingly common today, possibly because of sensitivities brought on by changes in how we grow and process food.

DIAGNOSTIC TESTS

Many of the tests I mention cannot be performed by general practitioners. If they do offer them, most will want to reserve testing as a last resort, relying on medications as a first option to suppress symptoms. Unfortunately, that's the way conventional medicine works. You may want to seek out a functional doctor by going to the website of some of the labs that process these tests and getting a list of practitioners who offer them in your area; try Genova Diagnostics or Verisana. Keep in mind, the practitioner offering these tests may not always be a medical doctor. Others, like chiropractors or those who are knowledgeable in the areas of nutrition and gut-related disorders, like myself, may offer them; these professionals may give you more holistic care and guidance than a conventional doctor can. These tests can vary in price, ranging from $150 to $800, not including the interpretation. Here are a few of the more important diagnostic tests that I recommend:

- **CELIAC AND GLUTEN SENSITIVITY BLOOD TEST:** This can help determine if you have celiac disease or gluten intolerance.

- **GI MAPPING OR A COMPREHENSIVE STOOL ANALYSIS WITH PARASITOLOGY:** This type of test will reveal levels of inflammation in the bowel, whether you have food sensitivities, and how well you absorb nutrition. It documents your whole microbiome and reveals any infective pathogens or yeasts that may be present, including a possible parasitic infection.

- **SIBO TEST:** This breath test will reveal whether you have an overgrowth of bacteria in your small intestine.

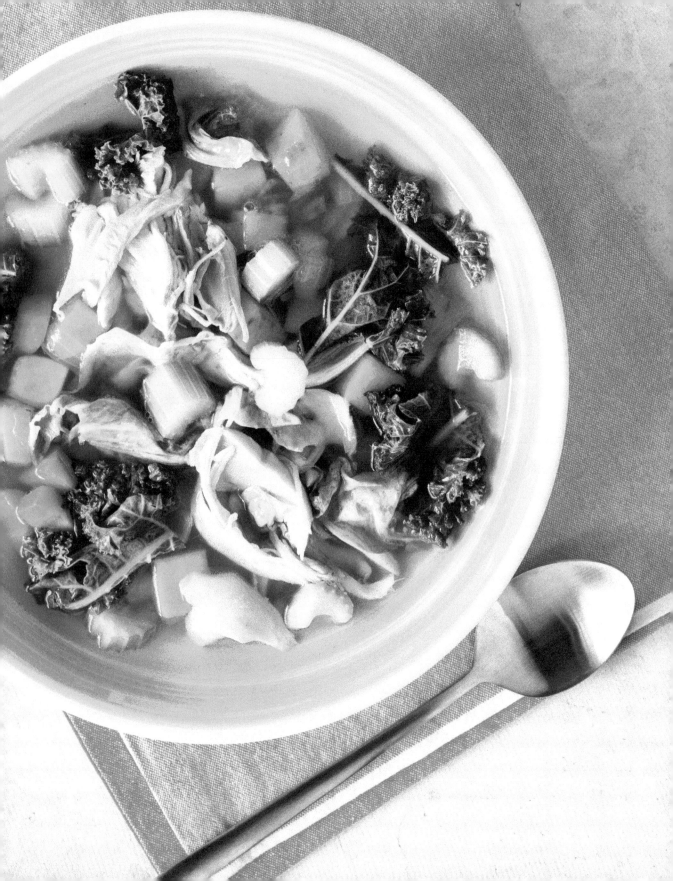

Healing Your Gut

Now that we know the overall role the gut plays in our health, it's time to talk about making some profound changes to help get things on track.

The Benefits of Good Health

The reality is that completely remediating a disturbed gut can take up to 2 years—and that's if you're diligent. The good news is that there are many changes you can make to help you begin experiencing relief from your symptoms right away that will also have a positive long-term impact on your imbalances. I also like to caution people who are not experiencing digestive distress or discomfort: It's very easy to assume that you are in the clear. But a disturbed gut does not always manifest as digestive distress; it can also affect your health in many other ways. Nourishing the gut is one of the most important things you can do for your overall health and well-being, including your immunity. I love it when my clients start working on their gut health and excitedly share that they are sleeping better, feeling more energetic, and experiencing better workout recovery time. I've even had women with infertility issues show up pregnant!

Good Nutrition

Growing up, I always looked forward to Sunday-morning breakfast with my family: eggs, bacon, toast, jam, pancakes, butter, syrup, and a big glass of orange juice. I also remember how miserable I would feel afterward. I would get a stomachache and congestion and couldn't keep my eyes open. I remember we would try to guess what might be causing my discomfort, but it never crossed our minds that it was what I had just eaten. My whole young life was spent that way, never making the connection between the Halloween candy and the chest cold, the chronic sinus infections and the sugary cereal after school, the daily stomachaches and the chocolate milk with lunch. Fortunately, people are starting to connect the dots and changes are happening. Simple, clean, homemade meals are crucial to overall wellness.

There are more specific changes you can make, too. There is no shortage of foods that are wonderful for your health, and the 4-week diet I detail will include most of them. But when it comes to nourishing the microbiome—literally feeding your beneficial organisms and starving out the bad ones—there are very specific foods for the job, and they happen to be delicious. In this book, you will become very familiar with prebiotic and probiotic foods, as well as specific grains, vegetables, and combinations of food that are not only very easy on the gut but help nourish the microbiota as well.

PREBIOTICS AND PROBIOTICS

If you've turned on your television or read a magazine or blog lately, you've probably heard of prebiotics and probiotics. These products are everywhere, and that's a good thing, because nothing could be more nourishing for your microbiome and overall health than including them in your daily routine. Historically, our diets were rich in probiotics and prebiotics, but sadly our modern diets tend to lack both.

PROBIOTICS are beneficial microbes naturally present in the soil and on the vegetables and fruits themselves. They're also present in all kinds of fermented foods, from milk to grains and beans to fruit, fish, and more. The process of preserving and fermenting cultivates beneficial microbes, making them almost 100 times more nutritious than regular foods.

PREBIOTICS is a fancy way of saying fiber, and fiber happens to be the food that beneficial microbes eat. I'll use my garden analogy once again—it is important to prune and water your garden, but if you don't fortify your soil with nutrients, your garden ecosystem will be in big trouble.

Commonly Suggested Diets for Gut Health

As you may have discovered in your quest to help fix your digestive issues, there are many diets that claim to heal the gut. Many are very effective but may be specific to a certain diagnosis. Here are a few of the more popular diets that you may have come across and what they are good for:

THE PALEO DIET was born from the idea that our ancestors led physically active lifestyles and ate only a high-quality diet of whole foods. Followers avoid processed foods, grains, most dairy, refined sugar, legumes, and vegetable oils. It is a good diet for weight loss and a good place to start for most people.

THE AUTOIMMUNE PROTOCOL (AIP) DIET is rooted in the Paleo diet but is far more restrictive and meant to reduce inflammation in the gut. It eliminates eggs, coffee, and all nightshades (like eggplants, peppers, or tomatoes) in addition to all the other "foods to avoid" on the Paleo diet.

It is designed for people with autoimmune issues like rheumatoid arthritis, lupus, and more.

THE WESTON PRICE DIET was inspired by Weston A. Price's research from the 1930s and is based on the traditional wholesome diet of our more recent ancestors. They were most likely farmers living off the land who ate seasonally and locally; they used the whole animal, including bones, healthy fats, and organ meats, and fermented and preserved fruits and vegetables. This diet holds that when our eating habits were complete and varied, we got better nutrition, as reflected in the low rates of noncommunicable diseases at the time.

THE LOW-FODMAP DIET helps reduce a class of carbohydrates called fermentable oligo-, di-, and mono-saccharides and polyols (FODMAPs) that are difficult for some people to digest. Many studies have shown that these carbohydrates could be responsible for a large percentage of IBS cases, which may develop into more severe issues like Crohn's disease when left untreated. A diet low in these carbohydrates has been proven to be very helpful.

THE BODY ECOLOGY DIET is a protocol developed by Donna Gates to combat yeast overgrowth and restore the body's "inner ecology." While the protocol was developed specifically to treat candidiasis, it has also been found to benefit the immune system as a whole. It eliminates all forms of sugar, including fructose from fruits. It also excludes grains that contain gluten.

THE GUT AND PSYCHOLOGY SYNDROME (GAPS) DIET is a therapeutic diet designed to heal leaky gut syndrome, reduce inflammation, and even treat certain neurological conditions. The plan removes refined carbohydrates and foods that are difficult to digest and swaps in foods rich in probiotics and nutrients to help give your gut health an upgrade.

FOODS TO ENJOY

These foods do not tax digestion and may even help heal the gut.

Essential Fats and Oils

The fats listed below are healing to the gut and excellent sources of essential fatty acids. Try to keep your unrefined oils away from sunlight and do NOT use them for cooking. Unrefined oils are rapidly damaged when exposed to sunlight and heat.

- Beef tallow or duck fat
- Coconut oil (unrefined)
- Ghee; unsalted grass-fed
- cultured butter (e.g., Kerrygold)
- Olive oil

Dairy and Dairy Substitutes

Most of the foods listed below are fermented, and none contain added flavors or sugars. Fermented dairy is very easy to digest and helps heal the gut and aid digestion by providing beneficial microbes.

- Kefir, either cow or goat milk (if store-bought, avoid flavored kefir with added sugar)
- Goat cheese
- Nut milks (especially homemade)
- Coconut and cashew yogurts

Fruits

Fruits with a low glycemic index are easier to digest and more supportive of your good gut bacteria.

- Blueberries
- Cranberries
- Goji berries
- Green apples
- Lemons
- Limes
- Mulberries
- Pomegranates
- Raspberries
- Strawberries

Vegetables

Most vegetables are excellent for gut health and digestion, though some people with advanced digestive issues can have trouble with them. Keep notes on what vegetables might be triggering digestive discomfort, and either make sure to cook those well or completely avoid those particular vegetables.

- Arugula
- Avocado
- Bamboo shoots
- Beets
- Broccoli
- Brussels sprouts
- Cabbage
- Carrots
- Cauliflower
- Celery
- Chives
- Cucumber
- Daikon
- Fermented vegetables
- Green beans
- Kale
- Lettuce (all varieties)
- Mushrooms
- Parsnips
- Peas
- Potatoes
- Radish
- Sea vegetables (all)
- Shallots
- Spinach
- Sprouts
- Squash
- Turnips
- Yams
- Zucchini

Vegetables high in prebiotic fiber: asparagus, dandelion greens, garlic, Jerusalem artichokes, leeks, onions, potatoes

Lacto-Fermented Foods

These foods can really jump-start your digestive health rapidly. Their healing ability surpasses that of any other food, and I encourage making a strong effort to include them. The fact that they are predigested by the bacteria takes the burden of digestion off your gut. Their nutritional value is 100 times what it was before being fermented, and the microbes help heal and seal the lining of the gut.

However, be cautious here: Some people with SIBO and histamine issues cannot tolerate fermented foods. I recommend trying small amounts of fermented foods after your first 4 weeks. There is always a period of bloating and gas when eating more fermented food; if the discomfort persists after five days, cross them off your list. If you can, though, your gut would benefit from adding these foods to your diet on a regular basis.

- Coconut kefir water
- Dairy kefir
- Cultured vegetables (such as kimchi or sauerkraut)
- Natto and miso

Grains and Grain-Like Seeds

These are the easiest options to digest because unlike gluten-containing grains, they are high in fiber, minerals, and vitamins and are very easy for the body to break down.

Soak grains for at least 24 hours, and then use bone broth to cook them, which helps digestion and absorption.

- Amaranth
- Brown rice
- Brown rice pasta
- Buckwheat
- Forbidden rice
- Millet
- Quinoa
- Quinoa pasta
- Spelt
- Tapioca
- Wild rice

Meats

Meats have excellent ratios of protein, fat, and micronutrients. However, because they are so dense, I always recommend taking digestive enzymes with them and having large portions of vegetables (especially fermented vegetables) to help with digestion. Bone broths help repair the gut lining and contribute to overall healing in the body.

- Organic and grass-fed beef, bison, or lamb
- Wild game
- Bone broths (page 78)

Poultry and Eggs

Eggs are a complete food, and like meat, they can be difficult for some people to digest. I recommend taking digestive enzymes supplements with all animal products to ensure optimum digestion and absorption of the amazing benefits these foods have to offer.

- Duck
- Eggs, any
- Quail
- Organic, free-range chicken
- Turkey

Seafood

Seafood is so good for the gut because of its high healthy fat content. These healthy fats are not only necessary for our second brain, the gut, but our first as well. Choose the lowest-mercury seafood whenever possible; you can learn more from Seafood Watch online.

- Anchovies
- Crab
- Flounder
- Haddock
- Mullet
- Oysters
- Pollock
- Sardines
- Scallops
- Squid
- Tilapia
- Trout
- Wild-caught salmon and shrimp

Nuts

Nuts have gut-loving healthy fats and are high in nutrients as well, but it is easy to overeat them and cause digestive issues. Always limit nut intake to one handful per day.

- Almonds and cashews, soaked and raw
- Brazil nuts
- Pecans
- Pistachios
- Walnuts

Seeds

Try to eat seeds raw; if necessary, you can lightly toast them yourself.

- Pine nut
- Pumpkin
- Sesame
- Sunflower

Spices and Condiments

These items are tricky to buy from grocery stores because so many gut-hating ingredients are hidden in them. Avoid preservatives, sugars, and unpronounceable ingredients. Stick to organic spices that come in smaller containers so you don't have a spice sitting around in your cupboard for months going stale.

- Allspice, ground
- Apple cider vinegar, raw (Bragg's)
- Cacao, raw
- Cardamom, ground
- Cayenne, ground
- Chili flakes
- Chipotle pepper, ground
- Cinnamon, ground
- Curry powder
- Garlic powder
- Nutmeg, ground
- Nutritional yeast
- Olive oil
- Rosemary, dried
- Sea salt and Himalayan salt, air-dried
- Sesame oil
- Sweeteners, like Lakanto, stevia, yacón
- Thyme, dried
- Vanilla extract and other baking extracts

FOODS TO EAT IN MODERATION

Although these foods aren't bad for you when eaten occasionally, when eaten in abundance they can hinder healing, create inflammation, and impair digestion.

Refined Oils

Limit to 1 teaspoon per day as a dressing.

Butter, commercially processed
Oils, refined

Dairy

Limit to ½ cup 3 times per week.

Cheese, hard, aged more
   than 1 year
Yogurt, plain and Greek, no
   sugar added

Fruits

Limit to 3 servings per week.

Apples, red
Bananas (½ a banana 2 times
   per week)
Dates

It's best to avoid juicing during this 4 weeks. All juicing should be done in moderation and only if you experience no digestive distress following consumption.

Vegetables

Limit to 2 servings per week.

Eggplant
Peppers
Potatoes, russet
Tomatoes

Grains

Limit to 2 servings per week.

Corn tortillas, non-GMO (only if
   you experience no digestive dis-
   tress after consumption)
Oats, gluten-free
Popcorn, plain, non-GMO
Tortilla chips, blue corn

Meat

Limit to 1 serving per week.

Beef, commercially raised
Lamb
Pork
Veal

Seafood

Limit to 1 serving per week.

Bluefish
Halibut
Light Tuna, canned
Sablefish (black cod)
Sea bass
Spanish mackerel, south Atlantic

Beans and Nuts

Limit to 1 cup per week.

Beans, home-cooked, pre-soaked
Macadamia nuts

Seeds

*Limit to 2 tablespoons, 2 times
per week.*

Flax
Chia
Hemp

Spices, Condiments, and Beverages

Limit to 1 serving 3 times per week.

Beverages, caffeinated (ideally, the
   goal is to eliminate caffeine)
Honey, raw
Tamari / soy sauce, gluten-free

FOODS TO AVOID

These foods can hinder healing, create inflammation, and impair digestion.

Fats and Refined Oils

"Butter" spreads, imitation
Canola or rapeseed oil
Corn oil
Fats, deep-fried
Fats, hydrogenated
Fats, trans
Margarine
Oils that have been heated to a
   smoking temperature
Safflower oil
Soy oil

Dairy

Buttermilk
Cheeses, non-aged
Cream, whipping
Creamers, nondairy
Half and half
Milk, condensed
Milk, pasteurized or nonorganic
Sour cream
Yogurts, flavored

Grains

Barley
Bulgur
Cereals, packaged
Chips
Cookies
Crackers
Oats, not gluten-free
Pastas
Rice, white
Wheat

Meats

Bacon, commercially packaged
Dried and cured meats with added
   nitrates and sugars
Hot dogs
Lunch meats
Processed meats
Sausages

Seafood

High-mercury seafood, like:

King mackerel
Marlin
Orange roughy
Shark
Swordfish
Tilefish

Beans, Legumes, and Nuts

Beans, canned with refined oils
Nuts, pre-roasted and salted
Peanuts and peanut butter
Soybeans

Seeds

Seeds, pre-roasted and salted

Spices, Condiments, and More

Agave alcohol: This has a high
sugar content and is damaging to
the digestive system.
Artificial sweeteners, like Splenda
and Sweet-n-Low
Caffeine: If you are sensitive to caffeine, avoid it completely on this
diet. Those who are not sensitive
should still limit their intake to
half a cup per day.
Energy drinks, diet drinks,
and soda
Foods that have been fried, over-
cooked, charred, or blackened
High-fructose corn syrup
Honey, pasteurized commercial
Ice cream
Juice, commercial and homemade:
Commercial juice is pasteurized
and has almost no nutrients; all
that's left is sugar. Homemade
juice can be hard on digestion
and is best avoided while healing
the gut. Also avoid kombucha
with added sugar. It's best to stick
to lacto-fermented beverages.

> **CONTINUED ON NEXT PAGE**

> **CONTINUED**

Ketchup, sauces, and dressings,
  commercial
MSG
Pastries
Salt, commercial iodized table,
  like Morton
Soy sauce

Store-bought products with
  added sugar
Sugar, refined and processed, like
  brown, coconut, palm, raw, etc.

General Tips

- **Use bone broth for cooking.** Bone broth (page 78) is nutrient dense and can aid in digestion. Use it to cook grains, stews, and vegetables and as a morning coffee substitute.

- **Buy a slow cooker.** Especially for those of you who are not handy in the kitchen, this gadget will change your life.

- **Carry your digestive enzymes.** Taking digestive enzymes can make a world of difference—but only if you are consistent about taking them at every meal. Carry them with you everywhere, and make it a habit.

- **Drink lemon water.** The juice of one lemon in a quart of room-temperature water can help upregulate digestion, alkalize your system, and hydrate your colon.

- **Eat slowly.** Take the time to relax and breathe when you eat. You cannot "rest and digest" if you are stuck in "fight or flight."

- **Manage stress.** Nothing disturbs your gut health more than stress. Make it your life's mission to find a way to slow down. There are many options for stress management. Some of my favorites are breathing techniques, mindful meditation, prayer, a short walk, or a 15-minute music break.

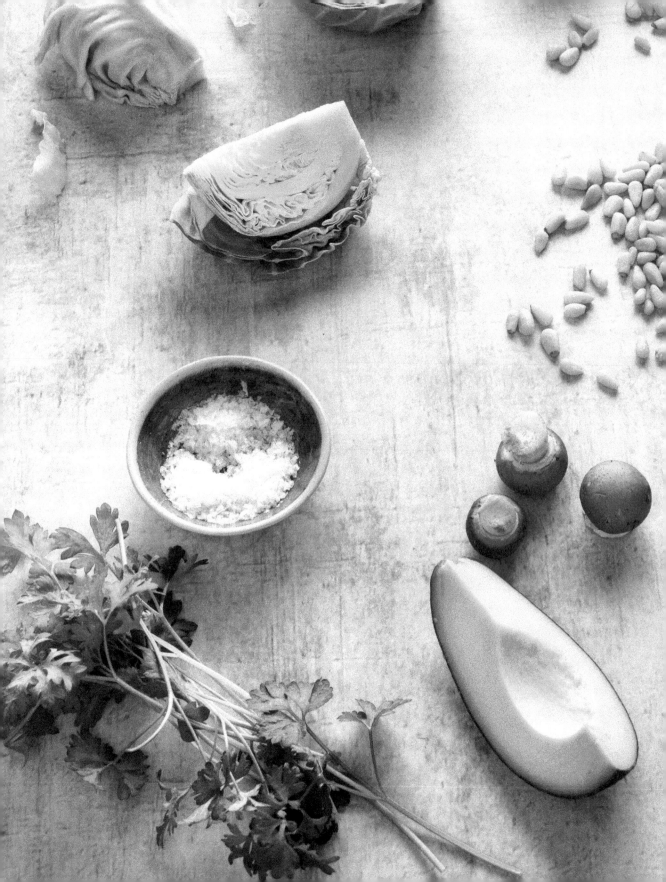

Rebuild and Plan for the Month Ahead

I cannot begin to express how profoundly important this chapter is. I have put thousands of clients—and family and friends—on diets over the last decade, and I can tell you with absolute certainty that the number one reason for failure is lack of preparation. I am guilty as well. We all know that excited feeling of starting a new diet. The first few days are amazing and then, after a hard day at work, you come home to realize you haven't prepared anything. So you do the easy thing and grab a frozen pizza, promising yourself you'll get back on track tomorrow.

To keep you from spiraling back into bad habits, in this chapter, I'll help you set yourself up for success, every step of the way.

Rebuild Your Kitchen

Think of your kitchen as a mechanic's garage. It won't operate well if it's in utter chaos; you'll spend half your time looking for misplaced tools, coping with items that are broken or old, or being frustrated at not having the correct tool for the job. The same is true for your kitchen. Putting things in convenient places, storing items correctly, and cleaning and sharpening your tools keeps you stress-free in the kitchen and makes it an enjoyable place to be. I remember hating to make stews because I was using my mother's slow cooker from the 1970s! It was a sentimental item that was keeping me from cooking healthier. Buying a modern slow cooker changed my life. Best of all, you don't have to break the bank to get a kitchen that works for you. Here are some tried and true tips.

The Pantry

Read labels on products, and get rid of anything that's highly processed, like rice cakes, chips, and other snacks. Toss products containing sugar, including high-fructose corn syrup, palm sugar, and the like. Also remove products that include vegetable oils like safflower and canola, added dyes, preservatives, or any chemical you can't pronounce.

Remove products that contain gluten, and look for sneaky gluten—even most soy sauces have gluten!

Eliminate roasted nuts and seeds, as the fats are damaged by high-temperature roasting and can be hard on the gut.

Now it's time to restock! Start by updating your spice rack, because spices equal flavor. At the very least, ensure you have these basics on hand:

- Bay leaves, dried
- Cayenne pepper, ground
- Cinnamon, ground
- Cumin, ground
- Curry powder
- Garlic powder
- Italian herb blend, dried
- Sea salt
- Vanilla extract

I like to save by buying in bulk, so I purchase good storage containers for grains, beans, nuts, and seeds, including opaque ones for storing high-fat nuts and seeds to keep them from going rancid. My bulk staples include:

- Almonds, raw, organic
- Flours, gluten-free (almond, coconut)
- Ghee
- Lentils and beans
- Millet
- Oats, gluten-free
- Oil, avocado
- Oil, coconut
- Oil, olive
- Pancake mix, gluten-free, sugar-free
- Pumpkin seeds, raw, organic
- Quinoa
- Sunflower seeds, raw, organic
- Tallow
- Wild rice

The Fridge

A clean fridge is a happy fridge. Take the time to remove everything and wash the shelves and produce bins.

- Remove condiments like soy sauce, ketchup, mayonnaise, and Worcestershire, BBQ, and teriyaki sauces.
- Remove old food containers and leftovers.
- Remove jams and jellies.
- Buy tamari, a gluten-free alternative to soy sauce.
- Use small mason jars to store homemade sauces, dressings, and nut milks.
- Buy unsalted butter (I like Kerrygold).
- Buy gluten-free miso paste (my favorite is Miso Master Organic Brown Rice Miso).

Take the time on Sunday to prep ingredients or cook components for the week ahead. I like to keep containers of:

- Chicken
- Quinoa
- Chopped veggies for soups
- Sliced veggies for snacks
- Small jars of dips for snacks
- Small jars of salad dressing
- Small jars of meat marinade
- Fermented vegetables
- Fermented dairy (or coconut kefir, if you aren't doing dairy)

The Freezer

Don't neglect your freezer; it deserves to be clean and organized as well. Pick up some freezer-safe containers to store leftovers or big-batch meals, and you won't need to turn to unhealthy quick fixes after a long day. Stock the freezer with those, plus:

- Mason jars of bone or veggie/mushroom broth
- Clean ice for smoothies
- Frozen berries
- Frozen bananas
- Leftover soups and stews for lunches and dinners

Cooking Equipment

Having the right tool for the job makes things almost effortless. I already mentioned my ancient slow cooker, and I want to reiterate how much an upgrade changed my life. These days, you can easily find coupons for home-goods stores; there's also Amazon or bulk shopping warehouses, like Costco, that can offer amazing deals on kitchen tools. You don't have to go broke creating the kitchen that works for you. I believe there are some items you should invest in higher quality for, but those can wait if it's not an option for your budget right now. I'll mention those below.

- **Slow cooker:** Many people are buying Instant Pots® these days, and I think those are fine, but I encourage you to use the slow cooker function. A single-purpose slow cooker will usually be much cheaper.
- **High-powered blender:** A Vitamix is a workhorse that you will use forever, but it's pricey, and the same job can be done with less-expensive blenders like NutriBullets, Ninjas, and Blendtecs.
- **A set of good kitchen knives:** Again, a high-quality chef's knife like a Messermeister will be a bit expensive, but you will use it forever. Still, the same job can be done with much less expensive knives; for the cost of one fancy German knife, you can buy a whole set of kitchen knives plus steak knives. Just be sure to get good ones—this is an area where quality does make a difference.
- **Cutting boards** for meats and vegetables
- **A large stock pot** for making bone broths and soups
- **A baking sheet**

- **A cast-iron skillet:** I find that I use my small cast-iron skillet for cooking meat often. It's not an absolute necessity, but it's nice to have if you are eating meat regularly.
- **Strainer and/or nut milk bag or cheesecloth** for making nut milks
- **A spiralizer and/or vegetable peeler:** While not strictly necessary (you can always cut your veggies into thin matchsticks or use a vegetable peeler to cut thin strips), spiralizers make it easy to create noodles out of your veggies!

Rebuild Yourself

A healthy diet is incredibly important for overall health, but it's not everything. According to several scientific studies, chronic stress is a main contributor to low stomach acid, ulcers, susceptibility to viral infection, and much, much more. Here are some important changes to consider incorporating into your life to help reduce stress and support yourself holistically.

- Maintaining a daily practice of meditation, prayer, or breath work
- Engaging in regular low-impact exercise, like yoga, power walking, or even ballroom dancing
- Reducing your electromagnetic exposure by turning off your Wi-Fi at night and putting your phone on airplane mode before bed
- Taking digestive supplements to ensure effective digestion, preventing food from sitting in your gut, rotting, and wreaking havoc on your microbiome. However, you must be careful with supplements—any preservatives or fillers may cause more harm than good. If you are going to use supplements, spend the money on getting the highest quality. Here are the supplements I don't leave home without:

  » A full-spectrum digestive enzyme with hydrochloric acid (HCL)
  » A spore-based probiotic like Just Thrive
  » A high-quality cod liver oil for adequate vitamin D and retinol
  » Grass-fed liver pills, particularly if you aren't a meat eater and don't mind supplementing
  » A high-quality multivitamin; Pure Encapsulations has great options

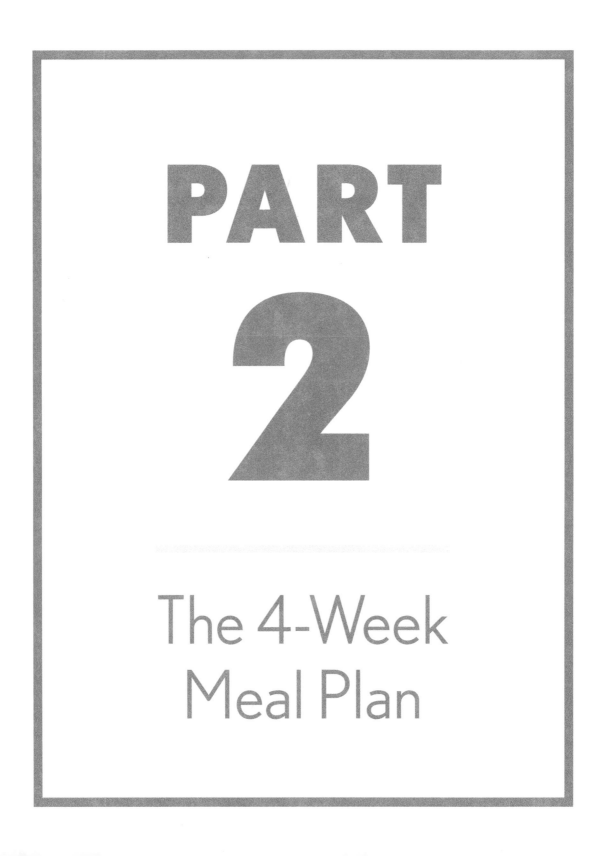

PART
2

The 4-Week
Meal Plan

This 4-week plan has been specifically designed with your success in mind. The foods on this diet were chosen because they are easy to digest, they are not on the list of foods that inflame and irritate the gut, and many of them help heal the digestive tract. The meal plan also incorporates leftovers to make your life easier and takes into consideration that it's not practical to cook three full meals a day. Specific cooking methods were chosen to make it easy to prepare a meal with the least amount of effort and the most amount of flavor. Breakfasts and lunches are designed to be "grab and go," so advance preparation is key.

I'll also provide you with practical tips to stay on track outside of your meal plan, such as during holidays, social events, vacations, and business travel. Finally, I'll help you transition off the 4-week plan with a whole chapter that eases you back into a normal but healthy diet.

As with any project, it is important to track your efforts. Sometimes progress can seem slow—until you look down at your journal and realize that more has changed than you thought. Jot down your favorite or least favorite part of each meal. What is easy, and what might be a more challenging part of the diet? Keep track of how you feel. Did you bloat after eating, or was this the first time you didn't bloat? Did a certain food cause a reaction? Do you have more energy at a certain time of day? How are your bowel movements? Were you consistent with drinking water and taking supplements? It's helpful to keep a record of everything, especially so you can reference your journal in the future to learn what worked for you and what didn't.

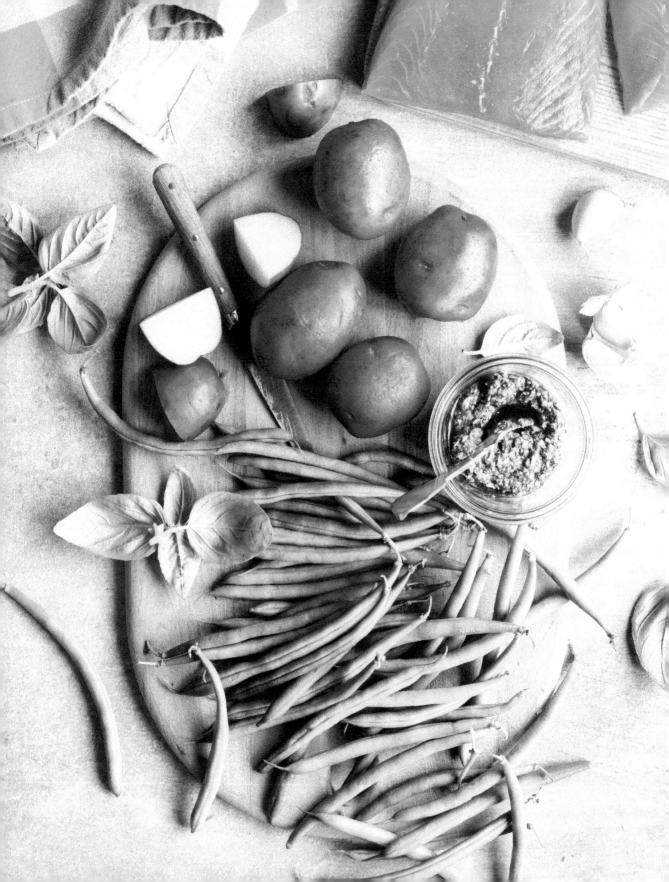

The Plan

After more than a decade of research and working with people with gut health issues, I am certain of a few things that promote success. The first is preparation; the next is consistency. Trying digestive enzymes a couple of times or taking a break from eating gluten for a few days will *not* make a dent in the damage done by years and years of eating a certain way. And the only way to truly be consistent is to have a plan in place. I don't know about you, but I am the type of person who likes someone to hold my hand through a new process. With that in mind, I've done just that: created a detailed plan that guides you through the process, holding your hand on this journey.

Week 1

Welcome to Week 1! I hope you are excited to embark on a healing adventure. This is always a rough week for everyone because change is hard. There's no easy way to get around that. However, all your preparation and the insight you will gain with the shopping guide and meal plans in this book should help ease any logistical issues that might arise. The more common challenges often involve side effects, hunger, and adjusting to a new routine. But I will reiterate that consistency is key. Habits are formed through repetition, and many of these new foods and daily routines will feel awkward and strange at first. Remind yourself that these new ways of preparing, cooking, and eating are medicinal, healing, nourishing—and life-changing. The benefits you gain will help you live a better, healthier life, so forge ahead and stick to the plan.

> **NOTE:** You should never experience a side effect or symptom that feels unbearable or intolerable; in particular, you should never experience vomiting, fever, bleeding, or severe pain. You should consult a medical doctor if any of these symptoms arise during this diet—or at any time.

WEEK 1 MEAL PLAN

	BREAKFAST	LUNCH	DINNER	SNACK
MONDAY	Quinoa Breakfast Bowl with Greens and Eggs (page 75)	Kitty's Chicken Soup (page 110) with 5-Ingredient Flatbread (page 163)	Grass-Fed Bison Quinoa Bowl with Turmeric-Ginger Sauce (page 128)	Green Apple Cashew Butter Bites (page 150)
TUESDAY	Leftover Kitty's Chicken Soup	Hearty Winter Salad with Forbidden Rice (page 84)	Green and Yellow Zoodles with Avocado Pesto Sauce (page 102)	Handful of raw mixed nuts, like almonds or cashews
WEDNESDAY	Avo, Ghee, and Radish Toast (page 71)	Hummus Vegetable Sandwich (page 87)	Baked Cod with Spinach and Capers (page 139)	5-Ingredient Flatbread and Hummus (page 163)
THURSDAY	Leftover Kitty's Chicken Soup	Leftover Baked Cod	Vegetarian Shepherd's Pie (page 95)	Digestive Tea (pages 157, 158)
FRIDAY	Blueberry & Seed Smoothie Bowl (page 66)	Leftover Shepherd's Pie	Cast-Iron Rib Eyes with Sweet Potato Fries (page 126)	Digestive Tea (pages 157, 158)
SATURDAY	Leftover Kitty's Chicken Soup	Pumpkin Seed Pesto Chicken and Arugula Sandwich (page 86)	Lemon Chicken and Roasted Baby Broccoli with Pine Nuts (page 115)	Frozen Yogurt Blueberries (page 154)
SUNDAY	Coconut-Bacon Waffles (page 73)	Leftover Kitty's Chicken Soup	Leftover Lemon Chicken Roasted Baby Broccoli with Pine Nuts	2 Almond-Coconut Haystacks (page 151)

I've mentioned preparation and planning many times throughout this book because they will be the keys to your success. Taking some time to sit down and decide exactly when you will execute your prep work is crucial, making your whole week a hassle-free breeze. In my household, Sundays are a big day for cooking, but you can choose any day that works for you. On this day, you'll spend several hours getting everything set for the week by following the detailed plans in this book (or, after the 4 weeks, choosing your week's worth of meals and planning what to make in advance). Each night during the week, make sure you set out a frozen meal in the fridge for the next day. Try these tips to make the most of your planning:

Sunday before your diet begins:

- Make fermented foods like sauerkraut or kefir at least 3 days before starting your diet.
- Make a big pot of Kitty's Chicken Soup (page 110), and freeze some for the week.
- Make some 5-Ingredient Flatbread (page 163) for the week.
- Spiralize your zucchini and refrigerate in an airtight container.
- Make enough Avocado Pesto Sauce (page 102) for several meals, and freeze half.
- Make enough hummus (page 87) for several meals, and freeze half.
- Freeze bananas for easy smoothies in the morning or on the go.
- Bake some chicken breasts, and freeze the extras. You can never have too many cooked or frozen chicken breasts.
- Make Green Goddess Dressing (page 164). Always have enough on hand to make a quick salad as a snack.
- Make some quinoa using a bit of the broth from the chicken soup you cooked.
- Pack your nuts in a resealable plastic bag, slice carrot sticks for extra snacks, and freeze your Frozen Yogurt Blueberries (page 154).
- Consider doubling the recipe amounts and freezing individual portions to make some recipes last all week. Example: Kitty's Chicken Soup (page 110).
- Make and freeze your Almond-Coconut Haystacks (page 151).

WEEK 1 SHOPPING LIST

Don't be intimidated: This will be the longest list in the book, as some items will last for the whole diet and are part of rebuilding your kitchen.

Canned and Bottled Items

- ☐ Apple cider vinegar, raw (I use Bragg's)
- ☐ Bone broth, 1 (32-ounce) carton (or homemade, page 78)
- ☐ Capers, 1 small jar
- ☐ Chickpeas, 2 (16-ounce) cans
- ☐ Coconut milk, light, 4 (16-ounce) cans
- ☐ Oil, coconut and olive, virgin
- ☐ Gluten-free soy sauce or tamari
- ☐ Tahini, 1 (16-ounce) jar
- ☐ Tart cherry juice, 1 (32-ounce) bottle
- ☐ Vegetable broth, 1 (32-ounce) box

Dairy, Eggs, Poultry, and Fish

- ☐ Chicken breasts, 4 (or more to cook and freeze)
- ☐ Chicken, whole, 1 (5-pound)
- ☐ Cod fillets (4)
- ☐ Eggs, large free-range (2 dozen)
- ☐ Ghee, or unsalted grass-fed cultured butter (I use Kerrygold)
- ☐ Greek yogurt, plain, 1 (16-ounce) container
- ☐ Milk (cow or goat), organic (1 gallon)

Meat

- ☐ Bacon, nitrate-free with no added sugar or maple syrup (1 pound)
- ☐ Bison, grass-fed, ground (2 pounds)
- ☐ Rib eye steaks, grass-fed, 2 (1-pound each)

Pantry Items

- ☐ Almonds, raw
- ☐ Baking powder
- ☐ Black pepper, freshly ground
- ☐ Bread, gluten-free (1 loaf)
- ☐ Cashew butter, preferably raw, 1 (16-ounce) jar
- ☐ Cinnamon, ground
- ☐ Coconut, unsweetened shredded, 1 (16-ounce) bag
- ☐ Coconut flour, 1 (16-ounce) bag
- ☐ Cranberries, dried, 1 (10-ounce) bag
- ☐ Cumin, ground

- [ ] Dark chocolate chips, unsweetened, 1 (16-ounce) bag (stevia-sweetened is fine)
- [ ] Dijon mustard
- [ ] Flaxseed, 1 (16-ounce) bag
- [ ] Flour, all-purpose, gluten-free (I use King Arthur)
- [ ] Forbidden or wild rice (Lundberg is my favorite)
- [ ] Granulated garlic or garlic salt
- [ ] Honey, raw
- [ ] Lentils, green (1 pound)
- [ ] Paprika (or Aleppo pepper, if you can get it)
- [ ] Pine nuts, raw
- [ ] Pumpkin pie spice blend, no sugar added
- [ ] Pumpkin seeds, raw and toasted
- [ ] Quinoa, 2 (16-ounce) bags
- [ ] Sea salt or Himalayan pink salt (make sure this is simply salt with no iodine, anticaking agents, or other ingredients)
- [ ] Tapioca flour, 1 (16-ounce) bag
- [ ] Tea bags, ginger and peppermint
- [ ] Turmeric, ground
- [ ] Vanilla extract

Produce

- [ ] Apples, green (4)
- [ ] Arugula, loose leaf, 1 (12-ounce) bag
- [ ] Avocados (3)
- [ ] Baby broccoli, or broccolini (1 bunch)
- [ ] Bananas (1 bunch, or more to freeze)
- [ ] Basil (1 bunch)
- [ ] Beet, yellow (1)
- [ ] Bell peppers, mixed colors (2 pounds)
- [ ] Blueberries (1 pint, or more to freeze)
- [ ] Broccoli (1 large crown)
- [ ] Broccoli sprouts 1 (60-gram) container
- [ ] Butternut squash (1 small)
- [ ] Carrots (1 pound)
- [ ] Celery (1 bunch or head)
- [ ] Cilantro, fresh (1 bunch)
- [ ] Cucumbers, Persian (2)
- [ ] Garlic (4 heads)
- [ ] Ginger (1 knob)
- [ ] Greens, mixed, 1 (16-ounce) bag
- [ ] Jalapeño pepper (1)
- [ ] Lemons (3)
- [ ] Limes (2)
- [ ] Mixed berries, frozen, 1 (16-ounce) bag
- [ ] Mushrooms, cremini, button, and shiitake (1 pound)
- [ ] Onions (5 pounds)
- [ ] Parsley, fresh (2 bunches)
- [ ] Peas, frozen, 1 (16-ounce) bag
- [ ] Pomegranate (1)
- [ ] Potatoes, Yukon gold or russet (2 pounds)
- [ ] Radishes (1 bag or bunch)
- [ ] Rosemary, fresh (1 bunch)
- [ ] Scallions (1 bunch)
- [ ] Spinach, fresh, baby (2 [16-ounce] bags, prewashed)
- [ ] Yams, garnet, or sweet potatoes (3 pounds)
- [ ] Zucchini, green and yellow (1 pound)

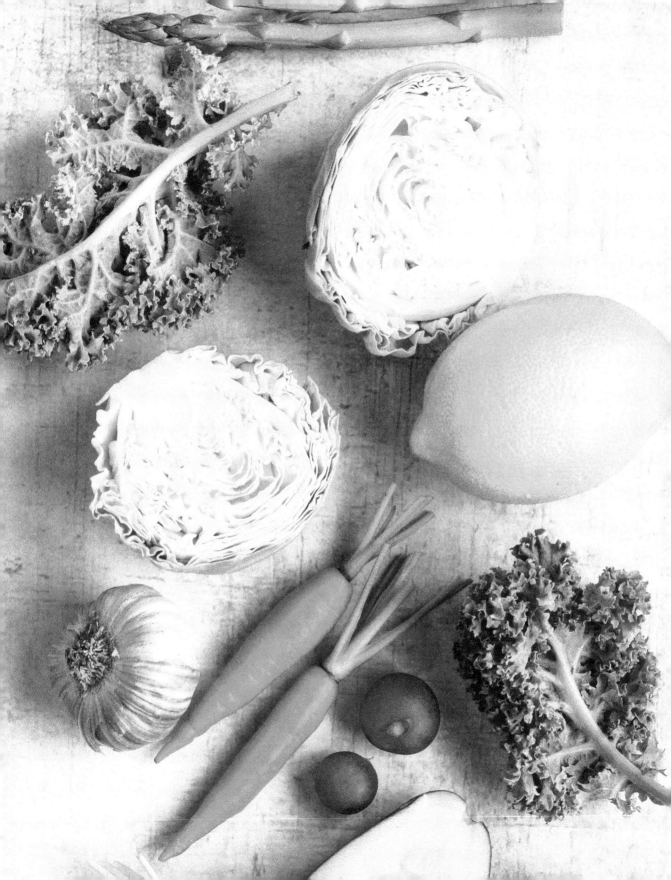

Week 2

By now your microbiome is getting the idea that these new changes might be permanent, and your beneficial bacteria are getting to work on important healing processes, like eliminating toxins from your blood and bowels. Some microbes are being eliminated because they don't belong, while others, like the fungus Candida, are dying off because they are no longer needed. Many people don't know that Candida is a yeast we all have in our bodies; it helps mitigate certain infections and issues like leaky gut. However, it can become unruly when a poor diet causes it to grow out of control, becoming an infection of its own. All these processes can cause a lot of changes in your body. For example, you might notice you've lost a few pounds but some skin conditions are worsening, or maybe you have more energy but seem a bit constipated. Try not to get caught up with why or exactly what is causing what. Simply be aware, write it all down, and stay the course.

WEEK 2 MEAL PLAN

	BREAKFAST	LUNCH	DINNER	SNACK
MONDAY	Mushroom & Beef Bone Broth (page 78)	Slow Cooker Kalua Pork and Cabbage (page 130) with Sauerkraut (page 167)	Roasted Vegetable and White Bean Salad (page 85)	Digestive Tea (pages 157, 158) and carrot sticks
TUESDAY	Ginger-Lemon Zinger Smoothie (page 67)	Leftover Roasted Vegetable and White Bean Salad	Leftover Slow Cooker Kalua Pork (page 130) with Carrot and Beet Coleslaw (page 83)	Green Apple Cashew Butter Bites (page 150)
WEDNESDAY	Leftover Kalua Pork with fried egg and leftover Sauerkraut	Green Goddess Cucumber Tea Sandwiches (page 88)	Chicken, Green Chile, Corn & Millet Casserole (page 119)	Carrot and celery sticks with hummus (page 87)
THURSDAY	Quinoa Breakfast Bowl with Greens, Eggs (page 75) and Green Goddess Dressing (page 164)	Chicken breast with mixed green salad and Green Goddess Dressing (page 164)	Leftover Chicken, Green Chile, Corn & Millet Casserole	Digestive Tea (pages 157, 158) and Green Goddess Cucumber Tea Sandwiches (page 88)
FRIDAY	Pumpkin Spice Smoothie (page 69)	Leftover Chicken, Green Chile, Corn & Millet Casserole	Hearty Winter Salad (page 84) and leftover Chicken Casserole	2 Almond-Coconut Haystacks (page 151)
SATURDAY	Avo, Ghee, and Radish Toast (page 71) with soft-boiled egg	Roasted Vegetable and White Bean Salad (page 85) with Green Goddess Dressing (page 164)	Grass-Fed Bison Quinoa Bowl with Turmeric-Ginger Sauce (page 128)	Veggie Spring Rolls with Miso Dipping Sauce (page 94)
SUNDAY	Coconut-Bacon Waffles (page 73)	Veggie Spring Rolls (page 94) with leftover Carrot and Beet Coleslaw	Vegetable-Coconut Curry Soup (page 81)	Digestive Tea (pages 157, 158) with a handful of nuts

WEEK 2 MEAL PREP

If you're feeling a little constrained, you can get creative, mixing and matching recipes from the book—there are endless combinations. When freezing food, make sure you label the items with a permanent marker or label maker. When you're getting ready for the week, go through your fridge and pantry; did you run out of anything? Write out your list for next week's meals. Here are some other prepping ideas to keep everything smooth and simple.

Sunday prep ideas:

- Make bone broth (page 78); freeze several quarts, and keep the rest in the fridge ready to use.
- Put the Kalua Pork (page 130) in the slow cooker.
- Cut carrot and celery sticks for snacks, and store in an airtight zip-top bag or container.
- Freeze bananas for quick smoothie options during the week.
- Make extra hummus (page 87) and freeze some.
- Make extra quinoa; it will last a week. It's a good go-to staple in case you run out of leftovers of something else that should've lasted longer than it did. When in doubt, there's always chicken breast and quinoa!
- Make the Chicken, Green Chile, Corn, & Millet Casserole (page 119) on Sunday; freeze half in individual containers.
- Make miso dipping sauce (page 94) in advance so you'll have enough on hand to toss with some quinoa or eat with carrot and celery sticks as a quick snack.

WEEK 2 SHOPPING LIST

Canned and Bottled Items

- ☐ Avocado oil
- ☐ Chickpeas, 2 (16-ounce) cans
- ☐ Corn, 1 (16-ounce) can
- ☐ Coconut milk, full fat, 2 (16-ounce) cans
- ☐ Green chiles, 1 (8-ounce) can
- ☐ Red curry paste (1 jar)
- ☐ Miso paste, brown rice, gluten-free (I like Miso Master)
- ☐ Tamari (gluten-free soy sauce) (1 bottle)
- ☐ White or cannellini beans, 1 (15-ounce) can

Dairy, Eggs, Poultry, and Fish

- ☐ Chicken breasts, boneless and skinless, 4 (or more to cook and freeze)
- ☐ Chicken thighs, boneless and skinless (2 pounds)
- ☐ Chicken, whole, 1 (5 pounds)
- ☐ Eggs, large free-range (1 dozen)
- ☐ Ghee, or unsalted grass-fed cultured butter (I use Kerrygold)
- ☐ Greek yogurt, plain, 1 (16-ounce) container
- ☐ Milk (cow or goat), organic (1 gallon)

Meat

- ☐ Bacon, nitrate-free with no added sugar or maple syrup (1 pound)
- ☐ Beef bones, including marrow bones (3 pounds)
- ☐ Bison, grass-fed, ground (2 pounds)
- ☐ Pork butt, bone-in (5 pounds)

Pantry Items

- ☐ Bay leaves, dried
- ☐ Kelp flakes (16 ounces)
- ☐ Millet, 1 (28-ounce) bag
- ☐ Nutritional yeast flakes, 1 (125-gram) container
- ☐ Porcini mushrooms, dried (2 cups, about 2 ounces)
- ☐ Rice paper wrappers (1 package), found in the Asian or international section
- ☐ Sesame seeds (12 ounces)

Produce

- ☐ Apples, green (6)
- ☐ Avocados (3)
- ☐ Bananas (1 bunch, or more to freeze)
- ☐ Basil, fresh (1 bunch)
- ☐ Beets (1 bunch)
- ☐ Bell peppers, mixed (1 pound)
- ☐ Broccoli (1 large crown)
- ☐ Butternut squash (1 small)
- ☐ Cabbage (1 small head, about 2 pounds)
- ☐ Carrots (1 pound; you may have some left from last week)
- ☐ Celery (1 bunch or head)
- ☐ Cucumber (1)
- ☐ Cucumbers, Persian (2)
- ☐ Dill, fresh (1 bunch)
- ☐ Garlic (you may have some left from last week)
- ☐ Ginger root, 2 (½-inch) pieces
- ☐ Greens, mixed, 1 (16-ounce) bag
- ☐ Lemons (2)
- ☐ Lettuce, romaine (1 head)
- ☐ Lime (1)
- ☐ Mushrooms, cremini, button, and shiitake (1 pound)
- ☐ Onions (2 large; you may have some left from last week)
- ☐ Parsley, fresh (1 bunch)
- ☐ Peas, frozen, 1 (16-ounce) bag
- ☐ Pomegranate (1)
- ☐ Potatoes, baby red (1 pound)
- ☐ Scallions (1 bunch)
- ☐ Spinach, fresh, baby, 2 (16-ounce) bags, prewashed
- ☐ Yams, garnet, or sweet potatoes (2 pounds; you may have some left from last week)
- ☐ Zucchini, green and yellow (1 pound)

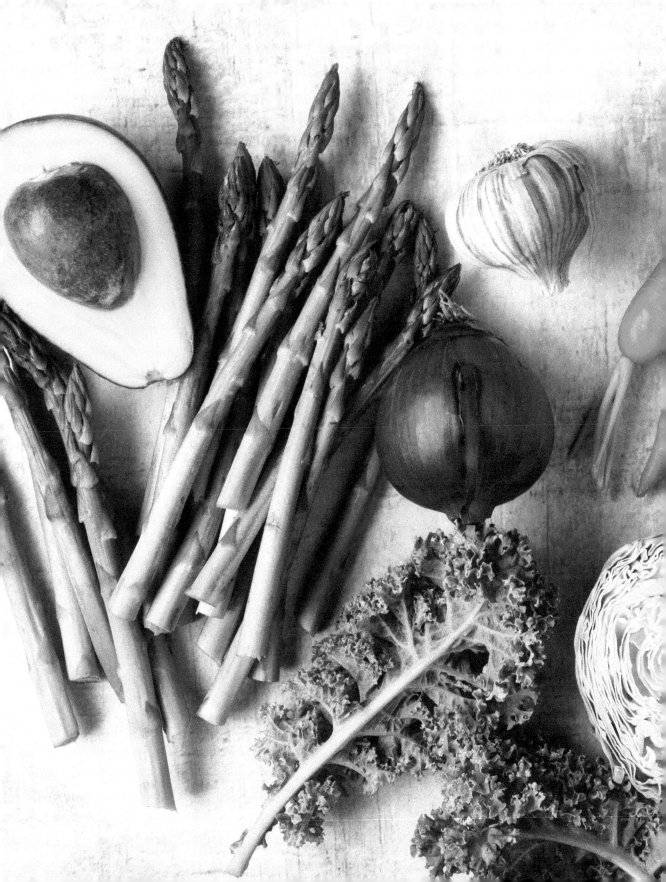

Week 3

Welcome to the halfway mark! You've done well and should pat yourself on your happy belly. But maybe your belly isn't completely happy yet, and you are getting discouraged because you see no major improvement. By now, your journal should thoroughly reflect your experiences with the food you are eating. Comb through it and identify if there might be foods on the list that you aren't quite ready for. The obvious culprits might be the fermented vegetables—many people will be used to them by now, but your unique body may not be ready yet. Maybe it's the chicken, eggs, beans, or dairy? These are also potential culprits. I like to keep in mind the image of the garden that you just tilled and replanted. You can't expect to walk out and see flowers blooming just yet. Be patient and observant, and try making some small tweaks to improve your comfort.

WEEK 3 MEAL PLAN

	BREAKFAST	LUNCH	DINNER	SNACKS
MONDAY	Ginger-Lemon Zinger Smoothie (page 67)	Leftover Vegetable-Coconut Curry Soup (from last week)	Mediterranean Slow-Cooked Chicken and Vegetables (page 118) and Cultured Blueberry-Coconut Pudding (page 153)	Digestive Tea (pages 157, 158)
TUESDAY	Chicken Liver Pâté on Seed Bread Toast Ends (page 106)	Leftover Mediterranean Slow-Cooked Chicken and Vegetables and Cultured Blueberry-Coconut Pudding	Spinach Fish Bake (page 144)	Digestive Tea (pages 157, 158)
WEDNESDAY	Leftover Chicken Liver Pâté on Seed Bread Toast Ends	Deviled Egg Salad (page 82) with 5-Ingredient Flatbread (page 163)	Leftover Mediterranean Chicken with Yams and Baby Broccoli with Turmeric-Ginger Sauce (page 98)	Greek yogurt and handful of almonds with chopped green apple
THURSDAY	Blueberry & Seed Smoothie Bowl (start Slow Cooker Mushroom and Onion Chicken [page 117] for dinner)	Leftover Chicken Liver Pâté on Seed Bread Toast Ends and leftover Cultured Blueberry-Coconut Pudding	Slow Cooker Mushroom and Onion Chicken	Frozen Yogurt Blueberries (page 154)
FRIDAY	Raspberry-Vanilla Smoothie (page 70)	Leftover Slow Cooker Mushroom and Onion Chicken	Zoodles with Lemon-Garlic Shrimp (page 141)	Ginger-Lemon Zinger Smoothie (page 67) and handful of nuts
SATURDAY	Avo, Ghee, and Radish Toast (page 71)	Pumpkin Seed Pesto Chicken and Arugula Sandwich (page 86)	Leftover Slow Cooker Mushroom and Onion Chicken	Digestive Tea (pages 157, 158); carrot and celery sticks and leftover Cultured Blueberry-Coconut Pudding
SUNDAY	Quinoa Breakfast Bowl with Greens and Eggs (page 75)	Hummus Vegetable Sandwich (page 87)	Halibut Fish Taco Bowl with Lemon-Cilantro Cream Sauce (page 142)	Bowl of Mushroom and Beef Bone Broth (page 78)

You should be getting the hang of things by now. You will probably notice that some dishes don't last as long as you thought they might, leaving you to rely on other items. Or maybe you had a lot more than expected. Remember, you can always run some hot water in the sink to thaw out frozen items at the last minute—that's part of why we prep extra on planning day! You will get better and better at meal prep the more you do it.

Sunday prep ideas:

- Start your Mediterranean Slow-Cooked Chicken and Vegetables (page 118) in the slow cooker.
- Make your Cultured Blueberry-Coconut Pudding (page 153), and refrigerate in an airtight container.
- Make your chicken liver pâté (page 106); freeze half and keep half in an airtight container in the fridge.
- Spiralize your zoodles (page 102), and refrigerate in an airtight container.
- Make your Seed Bread (page 162). You can also freeze half of this loaf.
- Boil eggs for Deviled Egg Salad (page 82).
- Make your Lemon-Cilantro Cream Sauce (page 142).
- Make sure you have enough frozen cooked chicken breasts on hand.
- Thaw out a container of leftover pumpkin seed pesto to use in lunches this week or make a new batch.

WEEK 3 SHOPPING LIST

Canned and Bottled Items

☐ Coconut milk kefir, 1 (12-ounce) bottle

Dairy, Eggs, Poultry, and Fish

☐ Chicken breasts, 4 (or more to cook and freeze)

☐ Chicken livers, organic (1 pound)

☐ Chicken thighs, organic, bone-in (2 pounds)

☐ Eggs, large free-range (2 dozen)

- ☐ Ghee, or unsalted grass-fed cultured butter (I use Kerrygold)
- ☐ Greek yogurt, plain, 1 (16-ounce) container
- ☐ Halibut fillets (8)
- ☐ Milk (cow or goat), organic (1 gallon)
- ☐ Shrimp, frozen or fresh (1 pound)

Meat

- ☐ Bacon, nitrate-free with no added sugar or maple syrup (1 pound)

Pantry Items

- ☐ Almonds, raw (12 ounces)
- ☐ Brandy, 1 bottle
- ☐ Bread, gluten-free (1 loaf)
- ☐ Cashew butter (1 jar)
- ☐ Flaxseed (10 ounces)
- ☐ Protein or collagen powder, vanilla flavor, 1 (10.4-ounce) container (I like Vital Proteins Vanilla & Coconut Water Collagen Whey Protein)
- ☐ Pumpkin seeds, raw (10 ounces)
- ☐ Sunflower seeds, raw (8 ounces)
- ☐ Walnuts, raw (16 ounces)

Produce

- ☐ Apples, green (4)
- ☐ Arugula, fresh, 1 (12-ounce) bag
- ☐ Avocado (2)
- ☐ Bananas (1 bunch, or more to freeze)
- ☐ Bell peppers, mixed (1 pound)
- ☐ Blueberries (2 pints)
- ☐ Carrots (1 pound; you may have some left from last week)
- ☐ Celery (1 bunch or head)
- ☐ Garlic (you may have some left from last week)
- ☐ Ginger, fresh (1 hand or knob)
- ☐ Lemons (2)
- ☐ Lettuce, romaine (1 head)
- ☐ Mixed berries, frozen, 1 (16-ounce) bag
- ☐ Mushrooms, cremini, button, and shiitake (1 pound)
- ☐ Onions, sweet (3)
- ☐ Parsley, fresh (2 bunches)
- ☐ Raspberries, frozen, 1 (12-ounce) bag
- ☐ Rosemary, fresh (1 bunch)
- ☐ Scallions (1 bunch)
- ☐ Shallots (4)
- ☐ Spinach, fresh, baby, 2 (16-ounce) bags, prewashed
- ☐ Thyme, fresh (2 bunches)
- ☐ Yams, garnet, or sweet potatoes (2 pounds; you may have some left from last week)
- ☐ Zucchini (4 large)

Week 4

We've entered the homestretch! How does it feel? At this point, most people are seeing drastic changes for the better. You're having more frequent, healthier bowel movements, less gas and belching, less bloating, and maybe no heartburn or abdominal pain. Or maybe you are experiencing subtle changes that you aren't consciously aware of. Don't overlook these small improvements, as they are signs of more to come.

Here are a few good signs to look out for:

- Gums no longer bleed when you floss.
- Dandruff is lessening or gone.
- Skin is starting to clear up or become less greasy around the nostrils or forehead.
- Less snoring and sounder sleep.

WEEK 4 MEAL PLAN

	BREAKFAST	LUNCH	DINNER	SNACKS
MONDAY	Miso Egg Drop Breakfast Soup (page 74)	Vegetable-Coconut Curry Soup (page 81)	Slow Cooker Beef Bourguignon (page 124)	Frozen Yogurt Blueberries (page 154) and Digestive Tea (pages 157, 158)
TUESDAY	Leftover Vegetable-Coconut Curry Soup	Chicken breast with mixed greens salad and Green Goddess Dressing (page 128)	Leftover Beef Bourguignon	Digestive Tea (pages 157, 158)
WEDNESDAY	Mushroom and Beef Bone Broth (page 78)	Leftover Beef Bourguignon	Lemon Butter Scallops over Wild Rice (page 146)	Digestive Tea (pages 157, 158)
THURSDAY	Ginger-Lemon Zinger Smoothie (page 67)	Leftover Mushroom and Beef Bone Broth and side salad with leftover Green Goddess Dressing	Feta Lamb Burgers (page 134) and side salad with leftover Green Goddess Dressing	Digestive Tea (pages 157, 158) and sliced green apples with cinnamon
FRIDAY	Avo, Ghee, and Radish Toast (page 71) with soft-boiled egg	Leftover Lamb Burger and side salad with leftover Green Goddess Dressing	Baked Cod with Spinach and Capers (page 139)	Digestive Tea (pages 157, 158) with Green Apple Cashew Butter Bites (page 150)
SATURDAY	Green Eggs & Ham (page 72)	Leftover Baked Cod	Quinoa Kibbeh with Lentils and Laban (page 132)	2 Almond-Coconut Haystacks (page 151)
SUNDAY	Coconut-Bacon Waffles (page 73)	Leftover Kibbeh with Lentils and Laban	Pesto Salmon, Green Beans, and Baby Reds (page 145)	5-Ingredient Flatbread (page 163) and leftover Laban

WEEK 4 MEAL PREP

Sunday meal prep:

- Start your Slow Cooker Beef Bourguignon (page 124).
- Make more bone broth (page 78) if you've run out.
- Make your Vegetable-Coconut Curry Soup (page 81). Freeze some and pack some for lunch.

WEEK 4 SHOPPING LIST

Canned and Bottled Items

- ☐ Bone broth, organic, 2 (32-ounce) cartons (or homemade, page 78)
- ☐ Burgundy red wine (1 bottle)
- ☐ Coconut milk, full-fat, 1 (16-ounce) can

Dairy, Eggs, Poultry, and Fish

- ☐ Chicken breasts, 4 (or more to cook and freeze)
- ☐ Cod fillets (4, about 2 pounds)
- ☐ Eggs, large free-range (2 dozen)
- ☐ Feta, sheep or goat milk (1 block, about 8 ounces)
- ☐ Ghee, or unsalted grass-fed cultured butter (I use Kerrygold)
- ☐ Greek yogurt, plain, 3 (16-ounce) containers
- ☐ Milk (cow or goat), organic (1 gallon)
- ☐ Salmon, wild-caught, 2 (1-pound) fillets
- ☐ Scallops, large sea, frozen or fresh (1 pound)

Meat

- ☐ Bacon, nitrate-free with no added sugar or maple syrup (1 pound)
- ☐ Beef bones, mixed, including marrow bones (3 pounds)
- ☐ Beef, stew meat, grass-fed (2 pounds)
- ☐ Ham steak, high quality with no nitrates or sugars added (4 to 6 ounces)
- ☐ Lamb, ground, grass-fed (4 pounds)

Pantry Items

- ☐ Allspice, ground
- ☐ Curry powder
- ☐ Oregano, dried
- ☐ Pine nuts, raw
- ☐ Porcini mushrooms, dried (2 cups, about 2 ounces)

Produce

- ☐ Apples, green (4)
- ☐ Avocado (2)
- ☐ Basil, fresh (1 bunch)
- ☐ Bell peppers, red and green (1 pound)
- ☐ Blueberries (2 pints)
- ☐ Cucumbers, Persian (3)
- ☐ Lemons (3)
- ☐ Lettuce, romaine (1 head)
- ☐ Mint, fresh (1 bunch)
- ☐ Mushrooms, cremini (10 ounces)
- ☐ Ginger, fresh (1 knob or hand)
- ☐ Green beans (1 pound)
- ☐ Parsley, fresh (1 bunch)
- ☐ Pearl onions, frozen, 1 (10-ounce) bag
- ☐ Potatoes, baby red (1 pound)
- ☐ Rosemary, fresh (1 bunch)
- ☐ Spinach, fresh, baby, 2 (16-ounce) bags, prewashed

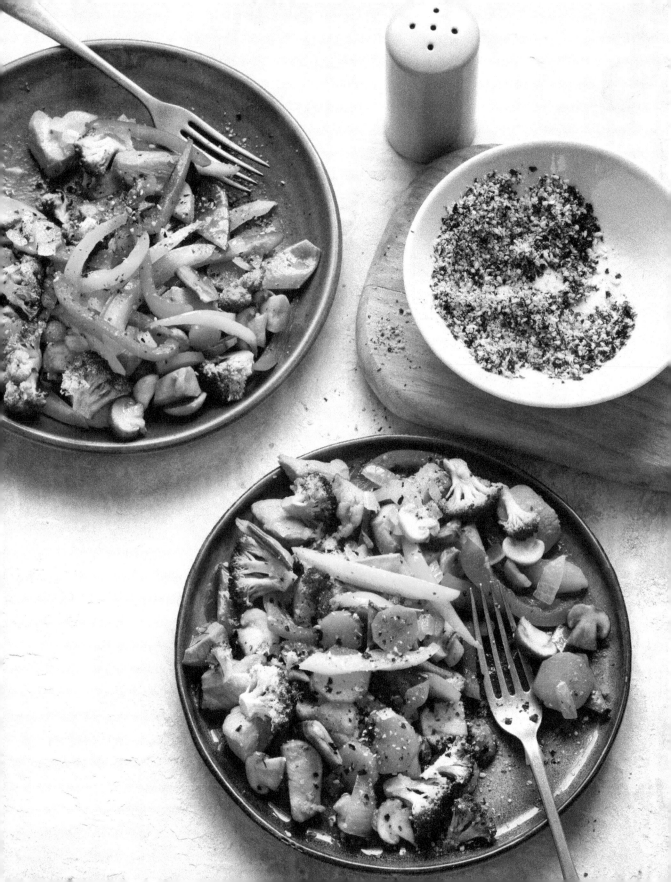

Beyond 4 Weeks

Congratulations on your massive accomplishment. It's truly something to be proud of—not only did you achieve your goal, but you have begun to shift your microbiome back into harmony. It is a scientific fact that even just 7 days of dietary changes can begin to alter the microbes in your gut for the better, but 4 weeks of targeted lifestyle and dietary changes can create exponential growth. You are now well on your way to better health.

If you are disappointed with your results, don't be; there are trillions of changes happening in your gut because of your healthy choices. No matter how significant your imbalances may be, these changes *will* start to shift the tides. If you are noticing massive changes, however, it might be tempting to go back to old habits—resist this temptation. Adding back one food every week is a good way to reintroduce old items. However, none of your food choices should include sugar, processed foods, or gluten. Instead, try adding some of the whole foods that are better in moderation, like tomatoes, or perhaps a vegetable or fruit juice. Be very aware of any symptoms that might be triggered by that food, like a runny nose or fatigue. In that case, you may need to avoid it a little longer.

Opposite: Chinese Garlic Chicken Stir-Fry, page 120

Holidays, Birthdays, and Social Events

Over my many years of dieting, I created my own special term for holidays, birthdays, and special events: *traps*. How many times did I start a diet, then go to a birthday party, and that was the end of my diet? I would eat something out of guilt, obligation, or sheer weakness and then say, "I will get back on track tomorrow." Of course, that never happened. It's normal—everyone does it.

How do you avoid the traps? Don't go? Stay home for the holidays eating a bowl of fermented vegetables by the fireplace all alone? Of course not. Here are my 5 tips to avoid traps:

1. Find out what's on the menu ahead of time. If it doesn't work with your diet, eat before you go.

2. Take healthy snacks of your own.

3. Make a healthy hors d'oeuvres plate to share and impress everyone. Before long, they'll want to know all about your new diet that features such yummy, healthy food.

4. Kindly refuse food that isn't on your menu. There's no need to brag about your diet unless asked—you can keep it simple. Here's my go-to way to decline:

   THEM: "Here, Kitty, have some delicious chocolate cake."

   ME: "That looks amazing, but I'm on a gut-healthy diet right now. Thank you."

   THEM: "Oh, come on. It's my birthday."

   ME: "I'm sorry. Someday soon I'll be able to eat whatever I want, but not right now."

5. Many holiday recipes can be altered to fit gut-healthy diets. Explore your options.

Restaurants

Restaurants are another tricky trap. I will be completely honest with you: Restaurant dining is my biggest weakness. I absolutely *love* eating out. I love being served, I love the choices, I love the ambiance and all the people enjoying themselves. It really is the one thing I have the hardest time with. The problem is, almost all restaurants use ingredients that will inevitably set your gut health back, like sugar, gluten, and processed products. So they're best avoided except for special occasions. Even with a busy lifestyle, there's no need to eat out or order in every night once you get the hang of planning and have delicious leftovers ready for you at home.

When I began to reduce my restaurant visits to once or twice per month, my gut thanked me and the savings were astronomical—so much so that my bank account took notice. For those times when you *do* choose to dine out, here are some tips on how to avoid bad-for-you restaurant food:

- Check out the menu online to learn what you can eat before you get there.
- Call and ask if they offer gluten-free or sugar-free options.
- Take your own condiments: Bring a small bottle of tamari for sushi or a small container of salad dressing.
- Some options may not be on the menu. Don't be afraid to inquire if they can sauté your fish in butter or coconut oil instead of canola oil.
- Opt for simpler dishes like chicken and vegetables instead of a dish with complex ingredients that are hard to digest.
- Always refuse the bread—it's another gut health trap. Ask for a side salad instead, with dressing on the side.
- Please be kind with your requests. There's nothing more annoying than a person with food restrictions who is rude.

Vacations

I always recommend planning your 4-week meal plan diet away from vacations or holidays. However, sometimes it cannot be avoided—especially if it means holding off on healing your gut. For some people, there is never a good time for a diet, so now is as good a time as any. Here are 5 ideas for how to stay stress-free about your dietary choices while making the most of your vacation.

1. Always take digestive enzymes with you, especially to places that have very different environments than you are used to. They help you digest unfamiliar food and fight foreign bugs. Hydrochloric acid, or HCL (which is in most digestive enzyme products), can literally keep you from getting food poisoning.

2. Bring small reusable shampoo-type containers filled with healthy condiments, like sea salt, tamari, and vinaigrette.

3. Explore the local farmers' markets and buy fresh local produce to snack on.

4. Use the same tips I gave you for restaurant eating when dining out. Don't be afraid to kindly ask your waiter if they can accommodate your restrictions. These requests are far more common today than ever before.

5. Opt for the room with the kitchenette or small fridge, and hit the grocery store before you check in to your hotel. Stock your fridge with the basics so you aren't eating every single meal out. As a bonus, you will have more money for sightseeing and activities.

Meals on the Go

Simplifying healthy, clean eating can be easy. Just keep in mind the basics, and you can create a delicious, gut-friendly meal quickly. Keeping it simple is key.

1. 80/20 rule + dressing, sauce, or topping

   80 percent of your plate should be vegetables

   20 percent of your plate should be animal protein OR a grain/legume protein like quinoa or lentils

   PLUS a tasty dressing or sauce

   Examples of some vegetable options (80 percent): kale, green beans, mixed greens, broccoli, arugula

   Examples of protein options (20 percent): turkey patty, lamb chops, lentils, chicken, ground bison

   Examples of dressing, sauces, or toppings (+): pumpkin seeds, tamari, vinegar, olive oil, avocado

2. Make sure the food is cooked in healthy fat, like coconut oil or cultured butter. Or you can add a healthy fat after cooking, like sliced avocado and pumpkin seeds.

PART
3

The Recipes

The recipes in this book are all geared toward high-quality, wholesome, homemade, fresh ingredients, organic and non-GMO whenever possible. Where applicable, you'll see one or more of these dietary labels, including Dairy-Free (DF), Nut-Free (NF), Paleo, Vegetarian, or Vegan, and the recipe tip labels Slow Cooker, Quick Prep (the meal doesn't require more than 10 minutes of preparation), and 5 Ingredients (for recipes containing no more than 5 ingredients, excluding water, fats [like oils or butter], sea salt, pepper, and vinegar). You won't see any Gluten-Free labels because all of the recipes in this book are free of gluten.

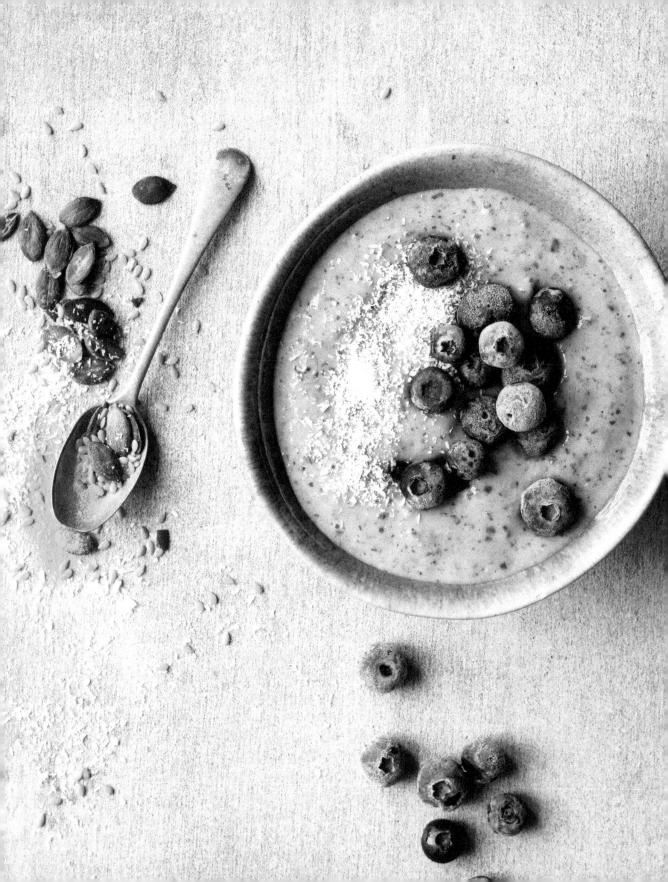

Breakfast and Smoothies

Opposite: Blueberry & Seed Smoothie Bowl, page 66

Blueberry & Seed Smoothie Bowl

Serves 1 | Prep time: 10 minutes | Paleo | Quick Prep | Vegan

I was introduced to smoothie bowls by my husband, who said they are quite a big deal in Brazil and, as it turns out, in Thailand, too. They are a nutritious, gut-friendly breakfast and a wonderful summer snack.

1 cup fresh, baby spinach

¼ cup mixed berries, frozen

½ banana, frozen

1 cup water or unsweetened nut milk or canned coconut milk

¼ teaspoon ground turmeric

½ tablespoon flaxseed

½ tablespoon raw pumpkin seeds

½ cup fresh blueberries

1 tablespoon unsweetened shredded coconut

1. In a blender, combine the spinach, frozen berries, banana, water, turmeric, flaxseed, and pumpkin seeds. Blend until smooth but not runny—it should be thick.

2. Pour the smoothie into a bowl, top creatively with fresh blueberries and coconut shreds.

Storage Note: Best consumed immediately.

Recipe Tip: Adding ice instead of water will keep the smoothie thick and cold.

Per Serving Calories: 254; Total fat: 12g; Saturated fat: 8g; Sodium: 32mg; Carbohydrates: 34g; Fiber: 8g; Protein: 6g

Ginger-Lemon Zinger Smoothie

Serves 1 | Prep time: 5 minutes | 5 Ingredients | Paleo | Quick Prep | Vegan

This bright, tart recipe is powerfully healing and soothing. It's a detoxifying smoothie that your gut will love you for.

½ inch fresh ginger
  root, peeled

¼ teaspoon ground turmeric

½ lemon

1 green apple, quartered

1 cup romaine lettuce

1 cup water or unsweetened
  nut milk or coconut milk

1 cup ice cubes

1. In a blender, combine the ginger, turmeric, lemon, apple, romaine, water, and ice. Blend on high for at least 1 minute.
2. Add more water and blend some more if the consistency is too thick for your taste. Pour into a glass and enjoy.

Storage Note: Best consumed immediately. You can store this smoothie in an airtight container after you make it, but it should be consumed within an hour for maximum flavor and health benefits.

Recipe Tip: This smoothie can be a powerful detoxifier, and you may feel some tummy rumbling after drinking it. Don't worry; that's completely normal.

Per Serving Calories: 137; Total fat: 1g; Saturated fat: 0g; Sodium: 6mg; Carbohydrates: 36g; Fiber: 7g; Protein: 1g

Coconut-Cinnamon Colada Smoothie

Serves 1 | Prep time: 5 minutes | 5 Ingredients | Quick Prep | Vegetarian

This refreshing, creamy smoothie tastes like a naughty dessert but has excellent gut health properties. The kefir is loaded with beneficial bacteria, the pineapple provides necessary enzymes, and the cinnamon can improve indigestion, flatulence, and heartburn and even helps balance blood sugar.

1 cup ice

1 cup frozen pineapple

¼ cup plain goat or dairy kefir

½ cup coconut milk, full fat

¼ teaspoon ground cinnamon, plus more for garnish

1. In a high-powered blender, combine the ice, pineapple, kefir, coconut milk, and cinnamon. Blend until smooth.

2. Pour into a tall glass, top with a dash of extra cinnamon, and enjoy.

Storage Note: This smoothie will keep, covered with a lid, for 24 hours in the fridge. Give it a good shake before drinking after storing. However, it's best consumed immediately.

Recipe Tip: This refreshing smoothie can be poured into ice pop molds and frozen for delicious summer treats.

Per Serving Calories: 382; Total fat: 30g; Saturated fat: 26g; Sodium: 43mg; Carbohydrates: 31g; Fiber: 5g; Protein: 5g

Pumpkin Spice Smoothie

Serves 2 | Prep time: 5 minutes | Quick Prep | Vegetarian

I finally jumped on the pumpkin spice train, and I don't want to get off! This smoothie will satisfy any pumpkin-spice-loving fanatic. It tastes like fall and is a gut soother, too.

½ banana, frozen

½ cup coconut milk, full fat

1 cup plain Greek yogurt

½ teaspoon pumpkin pie spice mix (no sugar added)

½ inch fresh ginger root, peeled

1 teaspoon raw honey

Sprinkle of cinnamon, for garnish

1. In a high-speed blender, combine the banana, coconut milk, yogurt, pumpkin pie spice, ginger, and honey. Blend for at least 1 minute.

2. Sprinkle with cinnamon, pour into 2 tall glasses, and serve.

Storage Note: Best consumed immediately. You can store in an airtight jar for a day; shake well before drinking.

Recipe Tip: I like to take a digestive enzyme when a smoothie has many ingredients, just in case. It's also not a bad idea to add high-quality protein or collagen powders to any smoothie for extra nutrition.

Per Serving Calories: 259; Total fat: 16g; Saturated fat: 14g; Sodium: 60mg; Carbohydrates: 18g; Fiber: 2g; Protein: 13g

Raspberry-Vanilla Smoothie

Serves 1 | Prep time: 5 minutes | 5 Ingredients | NF | Paleo | Quick Prep | Vegetarian

If I didn't tell you this was good for you, you'd never know it! It tastes like a decadent sherbet or a tropical cocktail: tangy, sweet, luscious—and gut healthy.

1 cup frozen raspberries

½ cup Greek yogurt

1 inch fresh ginger
　　root, peeled

1 cup ice

½ teaspoon vanilla extract

2 scoops vanilla protein or
　　collagen powder (I love
　　Vital Proteins vanilla
　　coconut collagen)

1 teaspoon raw honey

1. In a blender, combine the raspberries, Greek yogurt, ginger, ice, vanilla, protein powder, and honey. Blend for at least 1 minute, or until smooth.

2. Pour into a tall glass and enjoy.

Storage Note: Best enjoyed immediately. You can store in the fridge in an airtight container for a few days; shake well before consuming.

Recipe Tip: If you are not tolerating dairy well, you can use unsweetened coconut yogurt instead of the Greek yogurt here.

Per Serving Calories: 271; Total fat: 1g; Saturated fat: 0g; Sodium: 222mg; Carbohydrates: 29g; Fiber: 8g; Protein: 38g

Avo, Ghee & Radish Toast

Serves 1 | Prep time: 5 minutes | Cook time: 5 minutes | 5 Ingredients | NF | Quick Prep | Vegetarian

The avocado toast craze has taken over the nation, and it has taken me right along with it. This is such an easy, densely nutritious, and versatile meal. It also has the perfect crunchy/mushy ratio. That is, crunchy toast and soft, creamy, mushy avocado with a nice crunchy, fresh bite of radish to finish.

1 large ripe avocado, pitted

Sea salt

4 radishes, sliced into thin discs

½ lemon, juiced

½ teaspoon olive oil

Freshly ground black pepper

2 slices gluten-free bread (my favorite is Schär)

1 teaspoon ghee, at room temperature

1. Scoop the avocado flesh into a small bowl, and mash with a fork until creamy and smooth. Add a pinch of salt, and mix well.
2. In another small bowl, mix the radishes with lemon juice and olive oil, season with salt and pepper.
3. Toast the bread to desired crispness.
4. Liberally spread the ghee on the warm toast, then spread the avocado over the ghee.
5. Top with the marinated radishes and enjoy.

Storage Note: Best consumed immediately.

Recipe Tip: A soft-boiled egg is the perfect addition to this already delectable recipe.

Per Serving Calories: 451; Total fat: 35g; Saturated fat: 7g; Sodium: 156mg; Carbohydrates: 38g; Fiber: 13g; Protein: 5g

Green Eggs & Ham

Serves 2 | Prep time: 10 minutes | Cook time: 15 minutes | NF | Paleo | Quick Prep

No, the eggs aren't really green! But the luscious avocado sauce is. This healthy spin on eggs Benedict is filling but won't leave you bloated.

FOR THE SAUCE

1 avocado

4 tablespoons butter or ghee, melted

Pinch paprika

¼ cup freshly squeezed lemon juice

⅓ cup hot water

½ teaspoon sea salt, or to taste

FOR THE GREEN EGGS & HAM

1 ham steak, 4 to 6 ounces (a high-quality brand of ham will not have sugar and other unwanted ingredients added)

2 tablespoons coconut oil or ghee, divided

2 cups fresh, baby spinach

Sea salt

Freshly ground black pepper

4 large eggs

TO MAKE THE SAUCE

In a blender, combine the avocado, butter, paprika, lemon juice, water, and salt. Blend until smooth. You may need to add a little more water and blend again to get it to a desired "saucy" consistency. Set aside.

TO MAKE THE GREEN EGGS AND HAM

1. In a small skillet over medium-high heat, sear the ham steak until slightly browned and flavorful, about 3 minutes on each side. Set aside.

2. Heat 1 tablespoon of oil in the skillet. Add the spinach and sauté until wilted, 2 to 3 minutes; salt and pepper to taste. Set aside.

3. Add the remaining tablespoon of oil to the skillet. Crack the eggs gently into the pan, and gently turn when whites are firm, after about 3 minutes. Immediately turn off the heat once you flip them for an over-easy yolk.

4. Plate your spinach first. Then cut the ham steak in half and place each piece on top of the spinach. Top with your egg and plenty of sauce!

5. Sprinkle with paprika and serve.

Storage Note: Best consumed immediately. Sauce can be made in advance and stored in an airtight jar in the fridge for a couple of days, but you may need to add a bit of water to improve the consistency.

Recipe Tip: If you are a vegetarian, you can omit the ham and replace with more greens or even a cup of forbidden rice.

Per Serving Calories: 641; Total fat: 60g; Saturated fat: 31g; Sodium: 1,267mg; Carbohydrates: 10g; Fiber: 7g; Protein: 20g

Coconut-Bacon Waffles

Makes 4 to 6 waffles | Prep time: 5 minutes | Cook time: 20 minutes | Paleo | Quick Prep

I found the greatest waffle iron by Cuisinart and went on a waffle-making binge! Of all the amazing recipes I tried, this was my favorite. Crispy, tender with little bits of crunchy bacon, and dripping with melted butter—no syrup needed! Of course, if you don't have a fancy waffle iron, you can use a skillet to make this recipe into pancakes!

½ cup coconut flour

½ cup tapioca flour

Pinch sea salt

2 teaspoons baking powder

½ pound bacon with no nitrates, sugar, or maple syrup added, cooked, cooled, and chopped into small crumbs

1 cup unsweetened coconut milk or nut milk

4 large eggs

4 tablespoons melted coconut oil, plus more for greasing the skillet

1 tablespoon raw honey, melted

4 to 6 teaspoons butter, divided

1. In a medium mixing bowl, combine the coconut flour, tapioca flour, salt, and baking powder. Mix well.
2. Add the bacon crumbs, coconut milk, eggs, coconut oil, and honey, and mix until smooth.
3. Heat a waffle iron or skillet to medium-high heat.
4. Grease the skillet or iron with coconut oil.
5. Scoop up about 1 cup of batter, and pour onto the hot skillet or waffle iron. If using a skillet, flip each pancake when the edges begin to brown and bubbles form in the middle, after about 3 to 4 minutes. They are done when they are browned on both sides and the edges are slightly crispy.
6. If using a waffle iron, the waffles are done when they are crispy and browned.
7. Serve hot with 1 teaspoon of butter per serving.

Storage Note: Best consumed immediately. They will store well in an airtight zip-top bag once they are completely cooled.

Recipe Tip: For a nice addition, you could add a fried egg on top. Or try spreading the waffles with nut butter and rolling them up for breakfast on the go.

Per Serving (1 waffle) Calories: 484; Total fat: 37g; Saturated fat: 23g; Sodium: 819mg; Carbohydrates: 22g; Fiber: 9g; Protein: 19g

Miso Egg Drop Breakfast Soup

Serves 2 | Prep time: 5 minutes | Cook time: 15 minutes | 5 Ingredients | DF | NF | Quick Prep

This incredibly easy recipe leaves no excuses for skipping breakfast . . . or any meal! Once you try it, it won't be hard to get used to the idea of soup for breakfast. This miso is warm, nutritious, satisfying, and extremely good for the gut.

2½ tablespoons gluten-free miso paste

4 cups bone broth (homemade, page 78, or store-bought organic) or vegetable broth

2 large eggs

2 cups fresh, baby spinach

½ teaspoon Gomashio (page 172)

1. In a medium sauce pan over medium heat, melt the miso paste. Slowly add the bone broth, and simmer for 10 minutes.

2. Crack the eggs into a small bowl, then pour them into the miso soup, whisking constantly in one direction until the eggs turn into ribbons.

3. Add the spinach, and continue to stir until the spinach is very wilted, about 3 minutes.

4. Sprinkle with the Gomashio and serve immediately.

Storage Note: Stores in an airtight container in the refrigerator for 3 days. Freezes well. Take some with you for lunch in a thermos.

Recipe Tip: You can add other healthy veggies like chopped scallions, shiitake mushrooms, and bok choy to make this an even more satisfying meal.

Per Serving Calories: 189; Total fat: 36g; Saturated fat: 3g; Sodium: 1,147mg; Carbohydrates: 7g; Fiber: 2g; Protein: 19g

Quinoa Breakfast Bowl with Greens and Eggs

Serves 2 | Prep time: 10 minutes | Cook time: 30 minutes | NF | Quick Prep

When I started my healing journey, I had a difficult time with breakfasts. That is, until I started to look outside of the normal breakfast staples and turned to dinner and lunch ideas like soups and, in this case, quinoa. This warm, comforting, healthy breakfast bowl is delicious and, most important, easy to digest.

1 tablespoon ghee, plus more if needed

1 garlic clove, minced

2 cups fresh, baby spinach

1 cup bone broth (homemade, page 78, or store-bought organic)

2 large eggs

3 cups cooked quinoa

1 ripe avocado, pitted and sliced

1 teaspoon Gomashio (page 172)

Sea salt

Freshly ground black pepper

1. In a medium skillet over medium-high heat, melt the ghee.
2. Add the garlic and sauté for 1 minute before adding the spinach.
3. Pour the bone broth into the pan. Cover and cook until the spinach has wilted by half, about 2 minutes. Set aside.
4. Crack the eggs into the same skillet and fry, adding a bit more ghee if necessary to prevent sticking. Set aside.
5. Portion the quinoa into 2 bowls. Add the cooked spinach, and top each portion with a fried egg.
6. Top with the sliced avocado, season with a sprinkle of Gomashio and salt and pepper, and serve.

Storage Note: You can store this in an airtight container for a day. The egg won't keep long without losing flavor or getting rubbery, but you can pre-make the grain bowl and add a freshly cooked egg later.

Recipe Tip: I pre-make a big batch of quinoa each week and store in an airtight container in the fridge. It saves so much time, and you can warm it up quickly and add it to everything. Remember to use bone broth to cook your quinoa.

Per Serving Calories: 649; Total fat: 30g; Saturated fat: 7g; Sodium: 120mg; Carbohydrates: 76g; Fiber: 15g; Protein: 22g

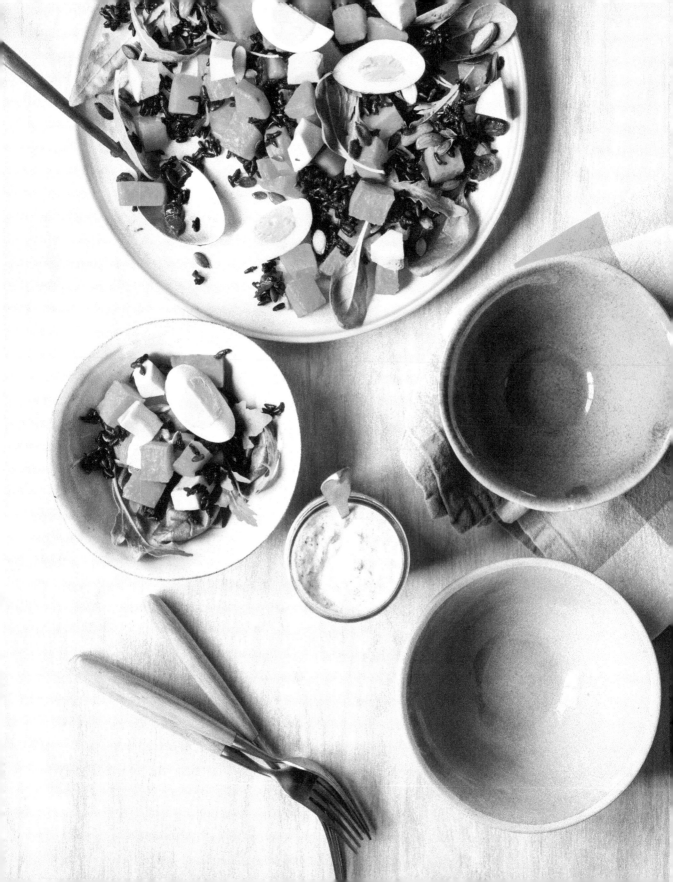

Soups, Salads, and Sandwiches

Opposite: Hearty Winter Salad with Forbidden Rice, page 84

Mushroom & Beef Bone Broth

Makes 2 to 3 quarts | Prep time: 45 minutes | Cook time: 37 hours | DF | NF | Paleo | Slow Cooker

A labor of love and healing, bone broth is probably the most nutritious recipe in this book. People have eaten this amazing food throughout history. Cooking bones to make soup was not only nutritious but an extremely clever way to maximize the whole animal and let nothing go to waste. The nutrients that leach out of the bones into the broth include collagen, glucosamine, hyaluronic acid, and minerals, all with strong gut-healing properties. And it is incredibly versatile in recipes. Make plenty; you are going to need it.

3 pounds mixed beef bones, ideally including marrow bones

½ cup dried porcini mushrooms

2 large carrots

1 large onion

2 celery stalks

1 dried bay leaf

2 tablespoons apple cider vinegar (I use Bragg's)

4 quarts water, plus more if needed

1. This is easiest to make in a large slow cooker (about 6 quarts). However, a large stock pot will do just fine—you will just have to keep an eye on it.
2. Preheat the oven to 400°F.
3. Place the bones on a baking sheet and roast for 30 minutes, until browned.
4. Roughly chop your mushrooms, carrots, onion, and celery.
5. Put the browned bones in the slow cooker or pot with the chopped veggies and the bay leaf and vinegar, and cover with the water.
6. Set your slow cooker on Low and cook for 36 hours. If using a pot, keep the heat very low and cover with a lid. Check the liquid level periodically, and add more water if too much is evaporating.
7. After 36 hours of simmering, remove the bones and place in a colander over a large bowl to catch the juices.
8. Pour the broth through a strainer into a large bowl. You will need to do this in batches, as the strainer fills up and needs to be emptied.
9. Discard the bones and vegetables. They are no longer nutritious—all the nutrients are in the broth.
10. Transfer the broth into mason jars for storage in the fridge or measure into freezer-safe containers or zip-top bags to store in the freezer.

Storage Note: Leave some space at the top of each container you intend to freeze so it will not break when the broth expands. Take one jar out of the freezer at night and place in the fridge to thaw; it will be ready to use in the morning.

Recipe Tip: The mushrooms are optional. I just love the richness they bring to the broth. The same recipe can be used with a chicken or turkey carcass or lamb, pork, or bison bones, as well. Use bone broth to make grains and beans, steam vegetables, make soups, or simply to sip instead of your morning coffee.

Per Serving Calories: 30; Total fat: 0g; Saturated fat: 0g; Sodium: 0mg; Carbohydrates: 1g; Fiber: 0g; Protein: 5g

Shiitake-Miso Cod Soup

Serves 2 | Prep time: 10 minutes | Cook time: 25 minutes | DF | Quick Prep

This soup is earthy, salty, hearty, and healthy. The miso adds depth of flavor and gut-friendly microbes from fermentation. Using bone broth makes it extra gut-healthy.

2 pieces fresh cod, about ½ pound total

1 tablespoon coconut oil

1 onion, sliced thinly

1 garlic clove, minced

1 inch fresh ginger root, peeled

4 or 5 fresh shiitake mushrooms, sliced thinly

16 ounces bone broth bone broth (homemade, page 78, or store-bought organic)

2 tablespoons gluten-free miso paste (I like Miso Master gluten-free brown rice)

1. Cut the cod into bite-size pieces.
2. In a large saucepan over medium heat, heat the coconut oil. Add the onion, garlic, and ginger, and sauté until the onion is translucent, 3 to 4 minutes.
3. Add the mushrooms, and sauté for 10 minutes, or until the mushrooms are tender.
4. Add the bone broth, and bring to a boil.
5. Add the miso paste, and stir until it has melted and fully incorporated into the soup.
6. Bring to a boil. Add the fish, and cook for 5 minutes, then turn off the heat and let poach for another 1 to 2 minutes.
7. Serve hot.

Storage Note: Store in the fridge in an airtight container for up to 4 days. Freezes well.

Recipe Tip: Adding other Asian ingredients into this soup can make it extra awesome. Try bok choy, scallions, or tofu.

Per Serving Calories: 259; Total fat: 9g; Saturated fat: 6g; Sodium: 1,056mg; Carbohydrates: 17g; Fiber: 4g; Protein: 29g

Vegetable-Coconut Curry Soup

Serves 2 | Prep time: 10 minutes | Cook time: 20 minutes | Quick Prep | Vegan

This aromatic soup is bright and tangy with ginger, but also creamy and comforting from coconut milk. It's a favorite in my house. It's versatile, stores well, and is easy to make ahead to take for lunches.

2 tablespoons coconut oil

2 garlic cloves, minced

1 inch fresh ginger root, peeled and minced

1 onion, sliced

6 cremini mushrooms, sliced

1 red bell pepper, chopped

1 green bell pepper, chopped

3 baby red potatoes, quartered

2 tablespoons curry powder

1 tablespoon red curry paste (optional)

2 tablespoons tamari (gluten-free soy sauce)

4 cups vegetable broth or bone broth for a non-vegan variation (homemade, page 78, or store-bought organic)

1 (16-ounce) can coconut milk

Sea salt

Freshly ground black pepper

5 fresh basil leaves, cut into thin ribbons

1. In a large pot over medium heat, melt the coconut oil. Add the garlic, ginger, and onions, and sauté until the onion is translucent, 3 to 4 minutes.
2. Add the mushrooms, red and green peppers, potatoes, curry powder, curry paste, and tamari, and stir until well combined.
3. Add the broth and coconut milk. Bring to a simmer for 15 minutes, or until the potatoes can be pierced easily with a fork.
4. Salt and pepper to taste. Ladle into 2 bowls, top with the basil, and serve.

Storage Note: You can make this ahead and store in the fridge in an airtight container. This soup also freezes well.

Recipe Tip: I like to squeeze fresh lime juice onto the soup before serving—it brightens the dish and brings out all the flavors and aromas. Feel free to add raw shrimp or raw chicken in the final 15 minutes of simmering.

Per Serving Calories: 915; Total fat: 69g; Saturated fat: 60g; Sodium: 1,068mg; Carbohydrates: 72g; Fiber: 17g; Protein: 16g

Deviled Egg Salad

Serves 3 to 4 | Prep time: 15 minutes | DF | Vegetarian

Here's a fun, yummy twist on an old-fashioned favorite. This salad is great to make in advance and have for lunch. Take the stress out of your next gathering by making a big bowl to bring to a party or picnic.

6 large hard-boiled eggs, peeled, cooled, and roughly chopped

¼ cup thinly sliced scallions, white and green parts

½ cup minced celery

1 red bell pepper, minced

1 tablespoon Dijon mustard

¼ cup Homemade Almond Mayo (page 166)

½ teaspoon paprika, plus more for garnish

Sea salt

Freshly ground black pepper

1. In a large bowl, combine the chopped eggs, scallions, celery, bell pepper, mustard, Homemade Almond Mayo, and paprika. Season with salt and pepper.
2. Mix well, adding more mayo if needed.
3. Sprinkle with a little extra paprika on top and serve.

Storage Note: You can make this ahead and store in the fridge in an airtight container for 1 week.

Recipe Tip: When hard-boiling eggs, I add a teaspoon of baking soda to the water before it boils, then let the eggs sit in cold water while I prep my vegetables to make them easy to peel.

Per Serving Calories: 225; Total fat: 16g; Saturated fat: 4g; Sodium: 237mg; Carbohydrates: 10g; Fiber: 1g; Protein: 12g

Carrot and Beet Coleslaw

Serves 2 | Prep time: 10 minutes | NF | Quick Prep | Vegetarian

This is one of my favorite healthy snacks. I always have some in my fridge. Crispy, fresh, and tart with a subtle sweetness, its prebiotics and probiotics are very gut-friendly.

3 large carrots, peeled and shredded (you can use a food processor or cheese grater)

2 large beets, peeled and shredded

1 large green apple, cored and shredded

1 tablespoon fresh dill, minced

1 tablespoon freshly squeezed lemon juice

¼ cup plain Greek yogurt

¼ cup toasted pumpkin seeds

In a large salad bowl, combine the carrots, beets, apple, dill, lemon juice, yogurt, and pumpkin seeds. Mix well and serve.

Storage Note: This salad keeps well in the fridge for a whole week in an airtight container.

Recipe Tip: You can use Homemade Almond Mayo (page 166) in place of the Greek yogurt to make this recipe vegan.

Per Serving Calories: 265; Total fat: 9g; Saturated fat: 2g; Sodium: 173mg; Carbohydrates: 41g; Fiber: 8g; Protein: 10g

Hearty Winter Salad with Forbidden Rice

Serves 4 | Prep time: 20 minutes | Cook time: 15 minutes | Vegetarian

This salad is a nice surprise thanks to the rice and tender yam bites. The nuts add a great crunch, and the dressing keeps it bright and light. It's gut-friendly and easy to digest.

2 yams, peeled and
   cut into cubes

2 tablespoons coconut
   oil or ghee

Sea salt

Freshly ground black pepper

1 ripe avocado, pitted
   and cut into cubes

½ cup dried cranberries

¼ cup sliced almonds

¼ cup toasted pumpkin seeds

1 bag mixed greens

1 cup forbidden or
   wild rice, cooked

¼ cup homemade Green
   Goddess Dressing
   (page 164)

1. Preheat the oven to 420°F.
2. On a cookie sheet, toss the chopped yams with the oil and spread evenly. Sprinkle with salt and pepper.
3. Roast for 15 minutes, or until tender and golden. Set aside to cool.
4. Once the yams have cooled, combine them in a large bowl with the avocado, cranberries, almonds, pumpkin seeds, greens, and rice. Toss with Green Goddess Dressing, mix well, and serve.

Storage Note: You can make this salad ahead and store in the fridge in an airtight container. Add the dressing when you're ready to eat.

Recipe Tip: Chicken or a hard-boiled egg is a delicious addition to this salad. Prepare all ingredients ahead of time so they are ready to toss together for a dinner party or after work for a quick meal.

Per Serving Calories: 392; Total fat: 21g; Saturated fat: 8g; Sodium: 31mg; Carbohydrates: 48g; Fiber: 9g; Protein: 8g

Roasted Vegetable and White Bean Salad

Serves 4 | Prep time: 15 minutes | Cook time: 10 minutes | NF | Vegan

This colorful dish is filled with flavor and is so packed with nutrients that you can eat it as a complete meal all by itself. But why stop there when you can throw on a grilled chicken breast or some slices of skirt steak? Who knew eating healthy was this colorful?

FOR THE SALAD

1 red bell pepper, cored and chopped into cubes

1 yellow bell pepper, cored and chopped into cubes

1 green bell pepper, cored and chopped into cubes

1 yam, peeled and cut into small cubes

1 cup cremini mushrooms, quartered

1 zucchini, cut into half moons

½ cup avocado oil

Sea salt

Freshly ground black pepper

1 (16-ounce) can white beans, rinsed

1 cup fresh, baby spinach

FOR THE DRESSING

¼ cup olive oil

¼ cup apple cider vinegar (I use Bragg's)

1 teaspoon nutritional yeast flakes

Sea salt

Freshly ground black pepper

1. Preheat the oven to 400°F.
2. On a large sheet pan, toss the bell peppers, yams, mushrooms, and zucchini with the avocado oil, and liberally sprinkle with salt and pepper.
3. Roast for 10 to 12 minutes, until everything is golden and tender.
4. Meanwhile, in a small bowl, make the dressing by mixing together the olive oil, apple cider vinegar, and nutritional yeast flakes. Season with salt and pepper to taste.
5. In a large bowl, mix the warm, roasted vegetables, beans, and dressing.
6. Lay the fresh baby spinach on the bottom of a large serving bowl, and serve the roasted vegetables on top of the spinach.

Storage Note: Best eaten immediately, but will keep for 2 days.

Recipe Tip: Beans can be hard on some tummies with advanced IBS or other types of digestive imbalances. I always recommend taking a digestive enzyme with meals to help with digestion, but some people may have to omit the beans to remain comfortable. Doing so will also make this meal Paleo.

Per Serving Calories: 392; Total fat: 17g; Saturated fat: 3g; Sodium: 237mg; Carbohydrates: 51g; Fiber: 15g; Protein: 12g

Pumpkin Seed Pesto Chicken and Arugula Sandwich

Serves 2 | Prep time: 10 minutes | Cook time: 35 minutes | DF | NF | Quick Prep

The secret to all chicken is the sauce or dressing, and this gut-friendly pesto is one of the best. The mineral-rich, bright pesto combined with the arugula makes this chicken pop. Make lots of extra pesto, and use it for dips for veggies and dressings for salads.

2 chicken breasts

1 tablespoon avocado oil

¼ teaspoon sea salt, plus more for seasoning

Freshly ground black pepper

3 garlic cloves, peeled and minced

1 cup fresh basil leaves, roughly chopped

1 cup fresh parsley, roughly chopped

½ cup pumpkin seeds

¼ teaspoon salt

¼ cup olive oil

4 slices gluten-free bread, toasted

1 cup arugula

1. Preheat the oven to 375°F.
2. Place the chicken breasts in a small baking dish. Drizzle with the avocado oil, and sprinkle with salt and pepper. Roast for 35 minutes, or until brown on top and cooked through. Set aside.
3. In a blender or food processor, combine the garlic, basil, parsley, pumpkin seeds, salt, and olive oil. Blend well, adding more oil if necessary to get a saucy, smooth, spreadable consistency.
4. Spread the pesto liberally on all 4 slices of bread, top with arugula and chicken before closing the sandwich, and serve.

Storage Note: You can pre-make the chicken and pesto and store in the fridge in an airtight container for 4 days.

Recipe Tip: You can skip the bread and simply top the chicken with the pesto as a sauce.

Per Serving Calories: 424; Total fat: 29g; Saturated fat: 6g; Sodium: 508mg; Carbohydrates: 25g; Fiber: 2g; Protein: 20g

Hummus Vegetable Sandwich

Serves 2 | Prep time: 25 minutes | Cook time: 5 minutes | NF | Vegan

Who doesn't love hummus? Add to that a host of crunchy fresh vegetables, and this sandwich is a hit.

1 (16-ounce) can chickpeas, drained, liquid reserved

2 tablespoons olive oil

3 garlic cloves, minced

½ teaspoon salt

¼ teaspoon freshly ground black pepper

3 tablespoons tahini (sesame seed paste)

2 teaspoons freshly squeezed lemon juice

¼ teaspoon ground cumin

¼ teaspoon paprika

4 slices gluten-free bread

1 Persian cucumber, sliced into thin discs

1 carrot, sliced into thin discs

1 cup broccoli sprouts

1. In a food processor or blender, combine the chickpeas, olive oil, garlic, salt, pepper, tahini, lemon juice, cumin, and paprika. While blending, slowly add 1 tablespoon of the reserved chickpea liquid to bring the hummus to a smooth consistency. Set aside.

2. Toast the bread, then liberally spread the hummus on all 4 slices.

3. Arrange the cucumber and carrot discs on the hummus, then add the broccoli sprouts.

4. Sprinkle with a bit of extra salt and paprika if desired, before closing the sandwiches and slicing to serve.

Storage Note: You can pre-make this sandwich the night before and store in the fridge in an airtight container. Hummus keeps in the fridge by itself for 1 week.

Recipe Tip: I serve this sandwich with a side of Carrot and Beet Coleslaw (page 83)—it's my favorite go-to lunch. The chickpeas and broccoli sprouts can cause some digestive distress, though. Cooking the beans yourself can help with that; soak dry chickpeas for 2 days, then simmer until tender. I also always recommend taking a digestive enzyme.

Per Serving Calories: 720; Total fat: 33g; Saturated fat: 7g; Sodium: 1,476mg; Carbohydrates: 93g; Fiber: 17g; Protein: 21g

Green Goddess Cucumber Tea Sandwiches

Serves 2 | Prep time: 15 minutes | NF | Vegetarian

I absolutely love afternoon tea in London. It is my favorite thing to do when I am lucky enough to be there. And the cucumber tea sandwiches are my favorite. But that cream cheese never fails to cause some bloating. Here is a healthy twist on a proper English classic.

1 ripe avocado, pitted

2 tablespoons freshly squeezed lemon juice

1 teaspoon minced fresh dill

1 garlic clove, peeled and minced

Sea salt

½ cup homemade Green Goddess Dressing (page 164)

2 Persian cucumbers, sliced into discs

4 slices gluten-free bread

1. Scoop the avocado flesh into a small bowl, and mash with a spoon until creamy.
2. Stir in the lemon juice, dill, garlic, and salt to taste.
3. In another small bowl, combine the Green Goddess Dressing with the cucumbers.
4. Spread some avocado mixture on each slice of bread, then arrange your dressed cucumber discs neatly atop before closing up the sandwiches. I like to use 2 layers of cucumbers for maximum crunch.
5. Slice into quarters, and serve with a cup of digestive tea. Keep that pinky up!

Storage Note: You can pre-make this sandwich and store in the fridge in an airtight container for 24 hours. You can also pre-make each item ahead of time and assemble prior to eating, in which case it will last for 4 days or so.

Recipe Tip: This is a great recipe to bring for baby showers, or as an appetizer at dinner parties.

Per Serving Calories: 357; Total fat: 18g; Saturated fat: 5g; Sodium: 781mg; Carbohydrates: 46g; Fiber: 9g; Protein: 8g

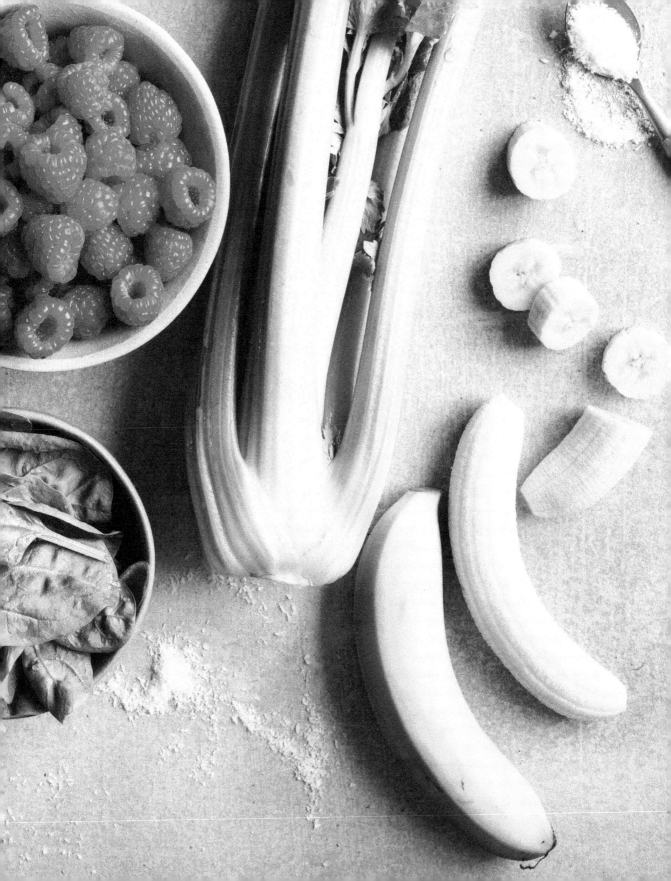

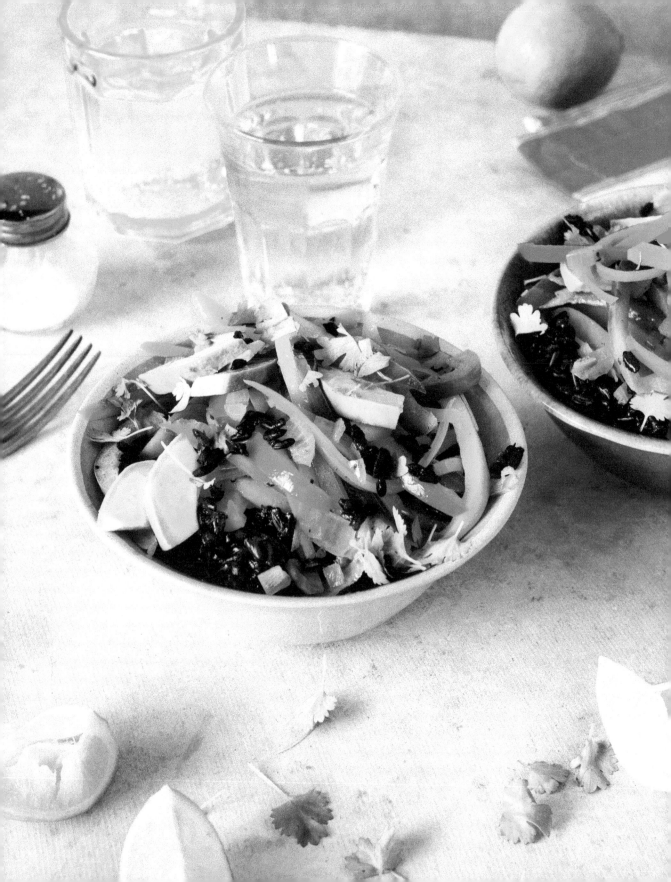

8

Vegetarian/Meatless

Opposite: Vegetable Fajita Bowl, page 100

Gut-Friendly Millet & Veggie Bowl

Serves 2 | Prep time: 10 minutes, plus overnight to soak | Cook time: 15 minutes | Vegan

Millet is a gluten-free grain that is incredibly easy to digest. It has a mild nutty taste that bursts with flavor, especially when combined with other bold, healthy ingredients.

½ cup millet, soaked overnight

1 cup vegetable broth

1 teaspoon sea salt, divided

2 tablespoons coconut oil

1 onion, diced

1 carrot, peeled and chopped

¼ teaspoon freshly
   ground black pepper

2 teaspoons freshly
   squeezed lemon juice

1 cucumber, chopped

1 (16-ounce) can kidney
   beans, drained and rinsed

1 tablespoon olive oil

Handful fresh mint leaves,
   cut into thin ribbons

1. Strain your millet, and put it in a saucepan. Add the broth and ½ teaspoon of salt to the pan, and bring to a boil. Reduce the heat to a low simmer and cover. Cook until the liquid has been absorbed and the millet is tender, 10 to 15 minutes. Make sure the heat is not too high and the millet doesn't start to burn. Set aside.

2. Meanwhile, in a medium skillet over medium-high heat, heat the coconut oil. Add the onion, carrot, remaining ½ teaspoon of salt, and the pepper. Cook until the onion is translucent, 3 to 4 minutes.

3. In a large bowl, combine the cooked millet and vegetables with the lemon juice, cucumber, beans, olive oil, and mint leaves. Add more salt to taste, if needed, and serve.

Storage Note: This dish will keep, refrigerated and covered with a lid, for 4 to 5 days. You can make a big pot of this in advance to add to other on-the-go meals.

Recipe Tip: This dish makes a great side or a main. It's also great with a fried egg on top for breakfast or lunch.

Per Serving Calories: 659; Total fat: 25g; Saturated fat: 14g; Sodium: 1,143mg; Carbohydrates: 91g; Fiber: 21g; Protein: 23g

Green Veggie–Stuffed Spaghetti Squash Bowl with Miso Dressing

Serves 2 | Prep time: 10 minutes | Cook time: 40 minutes | Quick Prep | Vegan

I used to be intimidated to cook with large squash. It seemed like a lot of work. But spaghetti squash changed all that for me. Now it's an easy go-to: filling, extremely healthy, and easy to digest. It can be mixed with just about everything and cooked in so many ways. This is one of my favorites.

FOR THE SPAGHETTI SQUASH

1 medium spaghetti squash, halved lengthwise and seeded

4 tablespoons coconut oil, divided

Sea salt

Freshly ground black pepper

2 garlic cloves, peeled and minced

1 bunch curly kale, stems removed, chopped into bite-size pieces

1 (16-ounce) bag fresh, baby spinach

½ teaspoon Gomashio (page 172)

FOR THE MISO DRESSING

2 tablespoons gluten-free miso paste

1 teaspoon toasted sesame oil

½ inch fresh peeled ginger root, grated (use a cheese grater or Microplane)

2 tablespoons apple cider vinegar (I use Bragg's)

2 tablespoons water

1. Preheat the oven to 400°F.
2. Liberally drizzle the inside of the spaghetti squash with 2 tablespoons of coconut oil. Sprinkle with salt and pepper.
3. Place the squash halves, cut-side down, on a foil-lined baking sheet. Roast for 40 minutes, or until you can pierce the squash easily with a fork. It could take longer, depending on the size of your squash.
4. Meanwhile, in a small jar, combine all the miso dressing ingredients and shake hard for 1 minute. Set aside.
5. In a large skillet over medium heat, heat the remaining 2 tablespoons of coconut oil and add the garlic. Sauté just until it turns slightly brown. Add the kale, and sauté for 4 minutes before adding the baby spinach.
6. Sauté until the greens cook down and are nicely wilted, about 3 more minutes.
7. To assemble your squash bowls, place one squash half on a plate and top with the cooked greens. Drizzle the miso dressing on top, and sprinkle with Gomashio. Repeat with the other portion.

Storage Note: To store squash, scoop out the flesh and keep in an airtight container with the cooked greens. Keep dressing separate. Dressing will keep in a jar in the fridge for 2 weeks.

Recipe Tip: This dressing can be made in larger quantities and used as a dip, salad dressing, or sandwich spread.

Per Serving Calories: 401; Total fat: 30g; Saturated fat: 24g; Sodium: 866mg; Carbohydrates: 29g; Fiber: 8g; Protein: 12g

Veggie Spring Rolls with Miso Dipping Sauce

Serves 4 | Prep time: 35 minutes | NF | Vegan

I used to absolutely love fried egg rolls but quit eating them for obvious reasons. And when I discovered spring rolls, I refused to try them out of respect for the original egg roll. But I gave in one day and was floored by how much better they were—and best of all, guilt-free. I thought I would miss the fried crunch, but made correctly, these have an even better crunch on the inside. They're pretty, too!

1 cucumber, spiralized into ribbon noodles or cut into thin sticks about 2½ inches long

1 carrot, julienned

1 red bell pepper, spiralized into ribbon noodles or cored and cut into thin sticks

1 ripe avocado, pitted and chopped

1 teaspoon sea salt

¼ teaspoon freshly ground black pepper

1 tablespoon freshly squeezed lime juice

4 rice paper wrappers or tapioca wrappers (find in any Asian food aisle, market, or online)

½ cup Miso Dressing (page 93)

1. In a large bowl, combine the cucumber, carrot, bell pepper, and avocado. Sprinkle with the salt and pepper, and drizzle with the lime juice. Mix well and set aside.
2. Soften the rice paper wrappers using a bowl of water. You can use your fingers or a paper towel to wipe each wrapper down with water until softened.
3. Scoop about one quarter of the veggie mix onto a wrapper. Cover the filling with one end of the wrapper, then fold in the sides and roll it up, just like making a burrito. Repeat with remaining wrappers and filling.
4. Serve with a side of Miso Dressing.

Storage Note: These will keep, refrigerated, in an airtight container for 4 days. Everything can be prepped in advance and stored in containers until ready to assemble.

Recipe Tip: Although this recipe calls for a spiralizer, you can also cut fine matchsticks with a knife or use a vegetable peeler to create thin strips. Serve the spring rolls cut in half as an appetizer at parties.

Per Serving Calories: 210; Total fat: 13g; Saturated fat: 2g; Sodium: 553mg; Carbohydrates: 24g; Fiber: 5g; Protein: 4g

Vegetarian Shepherd's Pie

Serves 4 | Prep time: 30 minutes | Cook time: 35 minutes | Vegetarian

We can all agree the best part of a shepherd's pie is not the traditional meat filling but the incredible comfort this casserole provides. You can have this quintessential comfort food in a totally vegetarian version. It is rich, grounding, filled with nutrition, and won't put you in a food coma.

FOR THE FILLING

1 cup green lentils, rinsed

4 cups vegetable broth, or as needed

2 tablespoons coconut oil

1 onion, diced

2 carrots, peeled and diced

1 cup frozen peas

1 red bell pepper, cored and diced

1 zucchini, chopped

1 cup broccoli, chopped into florets

FOR THE TOPPING

1 teaspoon sea salt, plus more for seasoning

4 cups water

2 pounds potatoes, Yukon gold or russet, peeled and quartered

⅓ cup plain Greek yogurt

2 tablespoons butter

Freshly ground black pepper

1. Preheat the oven to 450° F.
2. In a medium saucepan over medium heat, combine the lentils and enough broth to cover them fully. Bring to a boil, then lower to a simmer, cover, and cook until tender, about 20 minutes. Check regularly to make sure the liquid isn't evaporating too rapidly; simply add broth if needed.
3. Meanwhile, prepare the topping. In a large saucepan over high heat, bring the salt and water to a boil. Add the potatoes and boil until easily pierced with a fork, about 20 minutes. Strain the potatoes.
4. Use a fork or potato masher to mash the potatoes together with the yogurt, butter, and salt and pepper to taste. Set aside.
5. In a large skillet over medium-high heat, warm the coconut oil. Add the onion and carrots, and sauté until the onion is translucent, 3 to 4 minutes.
6. Add the peas, bell pepper, zucchini, and broccoli to the pan. Cook until the broccoli is tender but still bright green, 3 to 4 minutes. Remove from the heat.
7. Transfer the cooked vegetables and lentils to an 8-by-8-inch baking dish, and cover with the mashed potatoes. Pat the potatoes down with a spoon to form a casserole topping.
8. Bake for 10 minutes, or until the mashed potato topping starts to brown, and serve.

> **CONTINUED ON NEXT PAGE**

Vegetarian Shepherd's Pie

> **CONTINUED**

Storage Note: This dish will keep, refrigerated, in an airtight container for 4 days. I like to separate this into individual lunch-size portions for the week. It also freezes well.

Recipe Tip: Soaking the lentils for a few hours ahead of time can help reduce bloating and stomach discomfort. And, of course, taking digestive enzymes with meals is always recommended.

Per Serving Calories: 477; Total fat: 15g; Saturated fat: 10g; Sodium: 865mg; Carbohydrates: 69g; Fiber: 12g; Protein: 20g

Spaghetti Squash Fritters & Cucumber Laban

Serves 3 to 4 | Prep time: 30 minutes | Cook time: 30 minutes | 5 Ingredients | Paleo | Vegan

These little versatile bites of yumminess are easy to make, easy to eat, and easy on the gut. They can be appetizers, or served with a side of quinoa or a salad for a main dish.

1 large spaghetti squash (about 3 cups cooked)

¼ cup multipurpose gluten-free flour (I use King Arthur brand)

¼ teaspoon sea salt

Dash freshly ground black pepper

3 large eggs, beaten

2 scallions, white and green parts, chopped

1 tablespoon coconut oil

Cucumber Laban (see page 171)

1. Preheat the oven to 425° F.
2. Cook the spaghetti squash (see page 93). Let it cool, then scrape the flesh into a medium bowl.
3. Use a paper towel to wring out the squash. You want to get as much moisture out of the squash as possible. Set aside.
4. In a large mixing bowl, combine the flour, salt, pepper, and eggs. Mix well.
5. Stir in the squash and scallions.
6. Place a large skillet over medium-high heat. Heat the oil; it should be hot enough to nearly pop.
7. Using a spoon, scoop about ¼ cup of squash mixture onto the hot skillet and press down gently to flatten slightly. Cook until the edges stiffen and bubbles form in the center of the mixtures. Turn. Continue to cook until golden brown and crispy, about 1 to 2 minutes per fritter, per side. Repeat with the remaining squash mixture.
8. Serve with a side of Cucumber Laban (see page 171).

Storage Note: These will store in an airtight container for 3 days. The squash can be prepared in advance.

Recipe Tip: This dish is also great with a fried egg on top for breakfast or lunch.

Per Serving Calories: 192; Total fat: 10g; Saturated fat: 6g; Sodium: 248mg; Carbohydrates: 20g; Fiber: 1g; Protein: 8g

Yams and Baby Broccoli with Turmeric-Ginger Sauce

Serves 2 | Prep time: 15 minutes | Cook time: 1 hour | Paleo | Vegetarian

Honestly, you could put this sauce on a piece of cardboard and it would be amazing. But luckily, we aren't using cardboard today! Creamy yams and crunchy baby broccoli will be the vehicle for this tangy sensation. Your gut will thank you.

FOR THE VEGETABLES

2 large yams, scrubbed

1 bunch baby broccoli, or broccolini

1 tablespoon coconut oil

Sea salt

Freshly ground black pepper

2 teaspoons ghee

FOR THE TURMERIC-GINGER SAUCE

2 carrots, peeled

½ inch fresh ginger root, grated (use a cheese grater or Microplane)

2 teaspoons ground turmeric

¼ teaspoon sea salt

3 tablespoons cashew butter

¼ cup water, plus more if needed

FOR SERVING

Toasted pumpkin seeds

Gomashio (page 172)

1. Preheat the oven to 375°F.
2. Place the yams on a baking sheet and bake for 45 minutes to an hour, until you can easily pierce all the way through with a knife. Set aside to cool.
3. Meanwhile, make the sauce. In a blender, combine the carrots, ginger, turmeric, salt, cashew butter, and water. Blend until smooth and easy to pour, adding a little more water if it's too thick.
4. Place the baby broccoli on a baking sheet, and coat liberally with coconut oil, salt, and pepper. Roast for 25 minutes, or until the edges are browning and the stems are wilting.
5. Cut the yams in half, and scoop the flesh into a medium mixing bowl. Add the ghee, mix well, and season to taste with salt and a dash of pepper. Set aside.
6. Arrange the cooked baby broccoli in one side of a soup bowl. Next to them, place a few scoops of yams. Drizzle with the turmeric-ginger sauce, sprinkle with the pumpkin seeds and Gomashio, and serve.

Storage Note: The sauce will keep for 2 weeks in a jar in the fridge. It can be made in larger quantities and used for other dishes, salads, and dips. It may need a bit of extra water with each use, as it thickens over time. The yams can also be made in advance. The dish can be kept in an airtight container in the fridge for 3 to 4 days.

Recipe Tip: Fresh ginger keeps for up to 2 weeks unpeeled on the kitchen counter. You can also freeze it and grate it straight out of the freezer! Cut off half an inch to an inch at a time and peel with a spoon before using. A cheese grater or Microplane is the easiest, but watch your knuckles!

Per Serving Calories: 454; Total fat: 23g; Saturated fat: 11g; Sodium: 80mg; Carbohydrates: 56g; Fiber: 9g; Protein: 9g

Vegetable Fajita Bowl

Serves 2 | Prep time: 15 minutes | Cook time: 10 minutes | Vegan

This is such a quick, easy meal—and so nutritious and easy on the digestion. It's colorful, crunchy, and bursting with flavor.

2 tablespoons coconut oil

1 sweet onion, sliced thinly

1 large carrot, peeled into thin ribbons

1 garlic clove, peeled and minced

1 green bell pepper, cored and thinly sliced

1 red bell pepper, cored and thinly sliced

1 orange or yellow bell pepper, cored and thinly sliced

1 jalapeño pepper, seeded and minced (mild to no heat is best)

1 teaspoon sea salt

¼ teaspoon freshly ground black pepper

2 cups wild or forbidden rice, cooked

1 cup chopped fresh cilantro

1 lime, halved

1 small avocado, sliced

1. In a large skillet over high heat, heat the coconut oil. Add the onion, carrot, and garlic. Sauté until the onion is translucent, 3 to 4 minutes, taking care not to burn the garlic.

2. Add the bell peppers, jalapeño pepper, salt, and black pepper, and continue to sauté until the peppers are tender but still crunchy and vibrant, 3 to 4 minutes.

3. In a bowl, layer 1 cup of rice, top with half the vegetable fajita mixture, and sprinkle with ½ cup of cilantro. Repeat with the remaining portion.

4. Top with a squeeze of lime and the sliced avocado before serving.

Storage Note: This dish can keep for a couple of days in an airtight container in the fridge.

Recipe Tip: Everything can be sliced and chopped in advance and saved in containers in the fridge. Then it's ready for you to come home and throw it all together in minutes.

Per Serving Calories: 492; Total fat: 29g; Saturated fat: 14g; Sodium: 44mg; Carbohydrates: 61g; Fiber: 13g; Protein: 9g

Potato and Goat Cheese Gratin

Serves 3 to 4 | Prep time: 20 minutes | Cook time: 40 minutes | Vegetarian

This is a dish that I crave. It's creamy, cheesy, and true comfort food. When you have a hankering for mac and cheese, this is a wonderful, easy-to-digest substitute.

5 tablespoons butter

3 tablespoons gluten-free flour (like King Arthur)

1 teaspoon sea salt

2 garlic cloves, peeled and minced

2 teaspoons minced fresh rosemary

2 teaspoons minced fresh thyme

1 cup unsweetened nut milk (I use homemade almond milk)

8 ounces plain goat cheese

4 russet potatoes, sliced thin

1 cup gluten-free bread crumbs (I use Ian's Original)

1. Preheat the oven to 400°F.
2. In a saucepan over medium-high heat, melt the butter. Add the flour, and mix well.
3. Add the salt, garlic, rosemary, thyme, and almond milk. Bring to a simmer.
4. Add the goat cheese, and stir until it is melted.
5. In an 8-by-8-inch baking dish, lay out the potato slices one at a time to cover the bottom of the dish.
6. Pour a layer of cheese sauce over the potatoes.
7. Repeat, forming layers, until done.
8. Sprinkle the bread crumbs on top.
9. Bake for 30 to 35 minutes, or until the top turns golden brown, and serve.

Storage Note: You can store this in an airtight container for 3 to 4 days.

Recipe Tip: After slicing the potatoes, keep the slices in a bowl of cool water until ready to assemble. This keeps them from turning brown while you prep the rest of the dish. A mandoline is the easiest way to get a perfectly sliced potato, but it's not necessary—a knife works just fine.

Per Serving Calories: 555; Total fat: 31g; Saturated fat: 18g; Sodium: 1,296mg; Carbohydrates: 48g; Fiber: 4g; Protein: 20g

Green and Yellow Zoodles with Avocado Pesto Sauce

Serves 2 | Prep time: 15 minutes | Cook time: 5 minutes | NF | Paleo | Vegan

Spiralized vegetables are the best thing to happen to pasta for healthy people. While nothing truly compares to actual pasta, this recipe comes very close. The creamy avocado sauce wins the day; you'll want to put it on everything.

FOR THE ZOODLES

4 cups water

1 teaspoon sea salt

1 large green zucchini

1 large yellow zucchini

FOR THE AVOCADO PESTO

1 large avocado, pitted

1 garlic clove, peeled

Pinch sea salt

½ jalapeño pepper, seeded, mild in heat

1 tablespoon olive oil

½ cup chopped fresh cilantro

½ cup chopped fresh parsley

1 tablespoon freshly squeezed lemon juice

Water, if needed

1. In a medium saucepan, bring the water to a boil with the salt.
2. Using a vegetable spiralizer or a veggie peeler, spiralize both zucchini or peel into thin strips. Set aside.
3. In a blender, make the avocado pesto by combining the avocado flesh, garlic clove, salt, jalapeño, olive oil, cilantro, parsley, and lemon juice and blending until smooth. Add water by the tablespoon to get a smooth but not runny consistency, if needed.
4. Plunge the zoodles into the boiling water for 45 seconds, then drain immediately. Strain all excess water.
5. Divide the zoodles between 2 bowls, top each with half of the sauce, and serve.

Storage Note: The sauce will keep in an airtight jar for 3 to 4 days. Stir in a bit of lemon juice to reconstitute, if necessary. It's best to eat zoodles immediately or cook as needed. They don't store well cooked.

Recipe Tip: Spiralize veggies in advance and keep in an airtight container until you need them. This cuts preparation time down to almost nothing.

Per Serving Calories: 246; Total fat: 21g; Saturated fat: 3g; Sodium: 136mg; Carbohydrates: 15g; Fiber: 10g; Protein: 4g

Miso-Glazed Eggplant Kebobs with Cucumber Laban

Serves 4 | Prep time: 15 minutes | Cook time: 45 minutes | Vegan

As someone who has struggled with trying to be a vegetarian on and off, I discovered that the meals didn't seem complete to me the way an entrée with meat did. But there are a handful of filling, tasty vegetables that have a great texture. Eggplant is one of them. The side of Cucumber Laban really makes this dish a hit. (Laban is a Middle Eastern and Mediterranean yogurt sauce often served with meat dishes.)

3 medium eggplants, halved and cubed

1½ tablespoons coconut oil

Sea salt

Freshly ground black pepper

3 tablespoons gluten-free miso paste

1 tablespoon rice wine vinegar

1 teaspoon tamari (gluten-free soy sauce)

1 teaspoon toasted sesame oil

¼ teaspoon sea salt

2 teaspoons Gomashio (page 172)

2 cups Cucumber Laban (page 171)

1. Preheat the oven to 400°F.
2. Liberally coat the eggplant with coconut oil, salt, and pepper.
3. Slide the eggplant cubes onto 12 wooden or metal skewers (see recipe tip), leaving a small space between each.
4. Place on a parchment-covered baking sheet and bake for 30 minutes, or until browned and tender.
5. Meanwhile, in a small bowl, whisk together the miso, vinegar, tamari, sesame oil, and salt.
6. After 30 minutes, remove from the oven and brush the kebabs with the miso glaze, then return to the oven for 10 to 15 more minutes.
7. Sprinkle liberally with Gomashio, and serve with a side of Cucumber Laban.

Storage Note: Best eaten immediately, but will keep for 2 days. Cucumber Laban can be stored for 1 week.

Recipe Tip: Miso paste, rice wine vinegar, and tamari can be found in health food stores, Asian supermarkets, and online. Soak wooden skewers in cold water before using to keep them from burning. Use toothpicks instead of skewers for one-bite appetizers.

Per Serving Calories: 289; Total fat: 9g; Saturated fat: 6g; Sodium: 1,018mg; Carbohydrates: 36g; Fiber: 13g; Protein: 15g

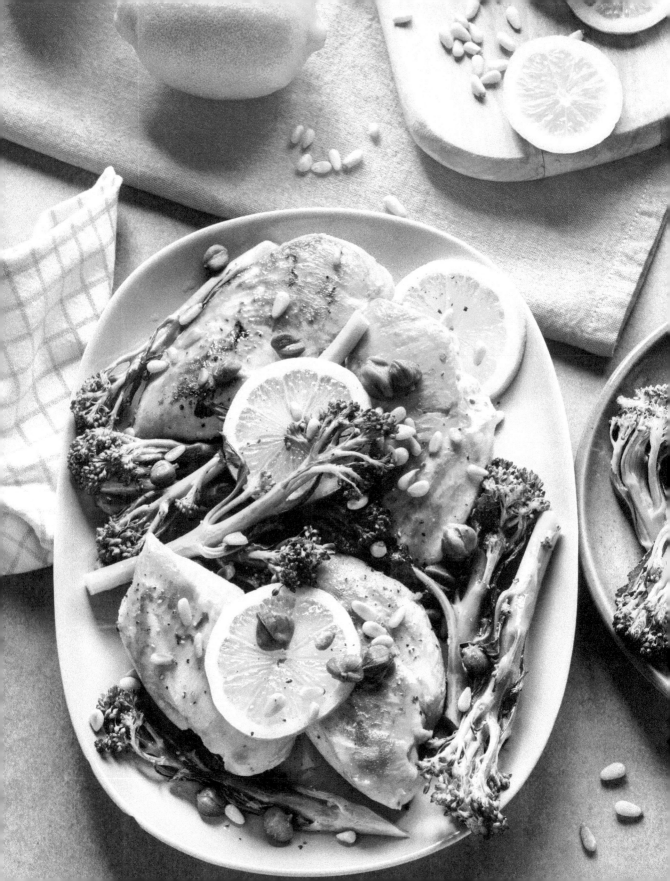

Poultry

Opposite: Lemon Chicken and Roasted Baby Broccoli with Pine Nuts, page 115

Chicken Liver Pâté on Seed Bread Toast Ends

Serves 4 | Prep time: 15 minutes | Cook time: 10 minutes | 5 Ingredients

If you aren't a fan of liver, your taste buds are about to change your mind. It's deliciously creamy, rich, earthy, and addictive. As if that weren't enough, this recipe is teeming with nutrition and gut-healing properties. Liver contains high levels of absorbable iron and folate, vitamin A, healthy fats, and all the B vitamins essential for a healthy gut and brain.

2 teaspoons salted butter, divided

1 shallot, minced

1 teaspoon minced fresh thyme

1 pound organic chicken livers, rinsed

1 teaspoon sea salt

½ teaspoon freshly ground black pepper

¼ cup brandy

4 slices Seed Bread (see page 162)

1. In a medium skillet over medium-high heat, melt 1 teaspoon of butter.
2. Add the shallot and thyme. Sauté until the shallot is translucent, 3 to 4 minutes. Transfer the shallot to a paper towel–lined plate.
3. Add the remaining teaspoon of butter, the chicken livers, salt, and pepper to the hot skillet. Sauté until the livers are lightly browned on all sides, 4 to 5 minutes total. Cut one open; it should still be slightly pink inside. Do *not* cook to well-done. Transfer to the paper towel–lined plate and set aside. Lower the heat to medium.
4. Carefully pour the brandy into the pan. You must use extreme caution when adding the brandy—it will ignite a flame, which is normal, but can be dangerous. The flame will die off as the alcohol is cooked down. After the flame has extinguished, use a spatula to deglaze the pan by scraping the brown bits off the bottom of the pan; this is where the flavor lives.
5. Once you've deglazed the pan, turn off the heat.
6. Let the chicken livers, shallots, and brandy cool for two minutes before transferring from the pan to a blender. Blend until completely smooth, at least 2 minutes.
7. Toast 4 slices of Seed Bread.
8. Cut the toast into bite-size pieces, spread liberally with the pâté, and serve.

Storage Note: Store the pâté in a small mason jar with a lid. It will keep for 1 week in the fridge and is usually eaten cold or at room temperature.

Recipe Tip: Some chicken livers do not come cleaned. If there are white stringy bits of sinew, you can use a pair of scissors or a sharp paring knife to cut them off.

Per Serving Calories: 803; Total fat: 66g; Saturated fat: 31g; Sodium: 1,325mg; Carbohydrates: 12g; Fiber: 6g; Protein: 40g

Sweet Potato Chicken Pie

Serves 4 | Prep time: 30 minutes | Cook time: 55 minutes | Paleo

This is such an easy recipe to make in large amounts and freeze for lunches. It's filling, with tons of healthy veggies and tender chunks of chicken. And the bone broth adds important gut-healing properties.

FOR THE TOPPING

2 large sweet potatoes, scrubbed

2 tablespoons butter

Sea salt

Freshly ground black pepper

FOR THE FILLING

2 tablespoons coconut oil or ghee

2 carrots, peeled and diced

1 onion, diced

4 cups bone broth (homemade, page 78, or store-bought organic)

2 pounds boneless, skinless chicken breasts, cut into bite-size pieces

1 cup frozen peas

1 red bell pepper, cored and diced

1 zucchini, chopped

1 cup broccoli, chopped into florets

1. Preheat the oven to 450°F.
2. Place the whole sweet potatoes on a baking sheet and roast for 45 minutes, or until you can slide a knife all the way through. This may take longer depending on the size of the sweet potatoes. Set aside to cool, leaving the oven on.
3. Meanwhile, make the filling. In a large skillet over medium heat, heat the oil. Add the carrots and onion, and sauté until the onion is translucent, 3 to 4 minutes.
4. Stir in the bone broth. Add the chicken breasts to the skillet, and bring to a simmer. Poach for 3 minutes.
5. Add the peas, bell pepper, zucchini, and broccoli. Simmer until the broccoli is tender but still bright green and the chicken is cooked through, about 5 minutes. Remove from the heat.
6. Cut the cooled sweet potatoes in half, and scoop into a mixing bowl. Mash with a fork or potato masher, mixing with butter and salt and pepper to taste.
7. Transfer the chicken and vegetable mixture to an 8-by-8-inch baking dish, and cover it with the sweet potatoes. Pat the topping down with a spoon.
8. Bake for 10 minutes, or until the sweet potatoes topping starts to brown, and serve.

Storage Note: This will keep, refrigerated, in an airtight container, for 4 to 5 days. I like to make a big batch and separate into individual lunch portions. It also freezes well.

Recipe Tip: Chop the veggies and bake the sweet potatoes in advance. With all the ingredients ready when you need them, this becomes a quick after-work meal.

Per Serving Calories: 506; Total fat: 16g; Saturated fat: 10g; Sodium: 283mg; Carbohydrates: 33g; Fiber: 7g; Protein: 59g

Kitty's Chicken Soup

Serves 4 | Prep time: 30 minutes, plus 20 minutes to cool | Cook time: 1 hour | DF | Paleo

I have been making this chicken soup for 15 years. Why? Because my husband is addicted. I make a massive pot of this, then freeze it so I have lunches for a whole week. Plus, there are many variations that keep it exciting, even after 15 years.

1 whole (roughly 5-pound) chicken without the gizzards, washed and patted dry with paper towels

1 tablespoon coconut oil, plus more for oiling the chicken

3 teaspoons sea salt

2 large carrots, peeled and cut into discs, then crescents

1 large onion, roughly chopped

3 celery stalks, chopped into crescents

3 garlic cloves, peeled and minced

1 yellow beet, peeled and quartered

1 small butternut squash, peeled, seeded, and chopped into bite-size pieces

2 quarts water

1. Preheat the oven to 400°F.
2. Place your chicken on a clean surface, and rub it down with oil. Then rub it with the salt.
3. Place the chicken in a baking dish and roast for 35 to 40 minutes. You will not cook it through, so depending on the size of the chicken, the time can vary. The skin will start to become golden brown, but the juice in the pan will still be pink. Remove from the oven and set aside.
4. Meanwhile, heat a large stock pot over medium-high heat, and add 1 tablespoon of coconut oil. Add the carrots, onion, celery, and garlic. Sauté until the onion is translucent, 3 to 4 minutes.
5. Add the beet and butternut squash, and cook for a few minutes, until slightly tender. Then add the water.
6. Bring to a boil, then carefully put the whole roasted chicken in the pot. If it's cool, simply use your hands. If it's hot, use tongs and a potholder. Keep the baking dish nearby.
7. Let the chicken poach in the soup for 10 minutes before carefully transferring it to the baking dish and lowering the heat to a low simmer.
8. Let the chicken cool for 20 minutes on the counter.
9. Once the chicken is cool enough to handle, move it to a cutting board and use a knife and fork to remove the meat. Close to the bone, you'll want to use your hands to get all the meat off.
10. Roughly chop the chicken with a knife, and return it to the soup pot for 2 to 3 minutes to warm through. Serve.

Storage Note: The soup will keep, refrigerated, in an airtight container for 4 to 5 days. It also freezes well. You can reserve the chicken carcass in a zip-top plastic bag, to make bone broth later; just pop it into the fridge.

Recipe Tip: For a variation, add 2 tablespoons of yellow curry to the first sauté of carrots, onion, and celery and add 1 can of coconut milk to the soup before adding the chopped chicken back in. Or try adding 2 cups of mixed mushrooms for a chicken mushroom soup. Switch up the veggies—try cabbage and kale. The possibilities are endless.

Per Serving Calories: 454; Total fat: 17g; Saturated fat: 7g; Sodium: 1,680mg; Carbohydrates: 19g; Fiber: 4g; Protein: 55g

Chicken Satay with NO-Peanut Sauce

Serves 4 | Prep time: 30 minutes, plus at least 6 hours to marinate | Cook time: 20 minutes | DF

These tender chicken bites are so addicting. The secret is in the marinade and how long you marinate the chicken. And why "NO-Peanut"? Peanuts are one of the top allergen-triggering foods; in fact, they might be number 1. And for this reason, we keep them away from the gut. But this nutty, exotic no-peanut sauce is even better than the original.

FOR THE CHICKEN

1 pound boneless, skinless
chicken breasts

FOR THE MARINADE

½ cup coconut milk

3 garlic cloves, peeled
and minced

1 teaspoon yellow
curry powder

½ teaspoon sea salt

¼ teaspoon freshly
ground black pepper

FOR THE SAUCE

1 tablespoon olive oil

3 garlic cloves, peeled
and minced

¼ cup creamy almond
or sunflower butter

1 tablespoon tamari

2 tablespoons toasted
sesame oil

1 tablespoon freshly
squeezed lemon juice

1. Slice the chicken into thin fingers.
2. Place the chicken fingers in a large zip-top bag with the coconut milk, garlic, curry powder, salt, and pepper, and seal well. Gently shake the bag to coat the chicken thoroughly. Place in the fridge for 6 hours or overnight.
3. Preheat the oven to 425°F.
4. Slide the chicken onto 10 to 12 wooden or metal skewers (see recipe tip), and place on a baking sheet.
5. Bake for 20 minutes, or until the chicken is cooked through.
6. Meanwhile, make the sauce. In a small saucepan over medium heat, heat the olive oil. Add the garlic, and sauté for 1 minute.
7. Add the almond butter, tamari, sesame oil, and lemon juice, and sauté, mixing well, for 3 to 4 minutes. Set aside.
8. Brush the chicken with the sauce before serving, serve it as a dipping sauce on the side, or both!

Storage Note: Both the chicken and sauce will keep, refrigerated, in airtight containers for 4 to 5 days.

Recipe Tip: If using wooden skewers, soak in cold water so they don't burn. I start mine soaking when I put the chicken in the fridge to marinate.

Per Serving Calories: 389; Total fat: 28g; Saturated fat: 9g; Sodium: 568mg; Carbohydrates: 7g; Fiber: 3g; Protein: 31g

Classic Roasted Chicken and Root Vegetables

Serves 4 | Prep time: 15 minutes, plus 10 minutes to rest | Cook time: 1 hour | 5 Ingredients

There's nothing like a Sunday roast with family or friends, and this one is always a favorite. But if you make it just for yourself, you'll have leftovers for days.

1 whole (roughly 4-pound) roasting chicken

1 tablespoon butter, at room temperature

4 tablespoons sea salt, divided

1 teaspoon freshly ground black pepper

4 garlic cloves, peeled, or 1 teaspoon garlic powder

2 yellow beets, peeled and quartered

2 turnips, peeled and quartered

2 parsnips, peeled, ends cut off, and halved

1 tablespoon coconut oil

1. Preheat the oven to 425°F.
2. Remove and discard the chicken giblets. Rinse the chicken well, and pat dry with paper towels.
3. Rub the chicken thoroughly with the butter. Liberally cover the chicken with 2 tablespoons of salt and the pepper. Don't forget to season inside.
4. Using a knife, make little holes in different parts of the chicken skin to slip the garlic cloves into, or sprinkle the garlic powder over the chicken.
5. Place the chicken in a baking dish, and roast for 1 hour. Check for doneness by cutting into the thickest part of the leg; the juice should run clear or the internal temperature should register 165°F on an instant-read thermometer. When it's done, remove from the heat.
6. About 40 minutes into cooking the chicken, place the beets, turnips, and parsnips on a baking sheet and drizzle liberally with the oil; sprinkle with the remaining 2 tablespoons of salt and mix so all the veggies are coated well.
7. Roast for 20 minutes, or until you can pierce the vegetables easily with a fork.
8. After the chicken has rested for 10 minutes, you can carve it, starting with the breast and working your way around.
9. Serve the chicken with the vegetables.

> **CONTINUED ON NEXT PAGE**

Classic Roasted Chicken and Root Vegetables

> **CONTINUED**

Storage Note: To store the chicken, you must remove the meat completely from the carcass. This is easier to do when cool. Then refrigerate the meat in an airtight container for 4 to 5 days. It also freezes well. The veggies can be stored with the chicken.

Recipe Tip: You can put the whole chicken carcass and giblets into a zip-top plastic bag, and toss in the freezer to make bone broth later. See page 78 for a bone broth recipe that adapts well to chicken.

Per Serving Calories: 293; Total fat: 12g; Saturated fat: 6g; Sodium: 4,774mg; Carbohydrates: 22g; Fiber: 6g; Protein: 24g

Lemon Chicken and Roasted Baby Broccoli with Pine Nuts

Serves 2 | Prep time: 10 minutes | Cook time: 30 minutes | Quick Prep

I make this lemony dish often because it's easy and stores well for lunches or fast dinners. I love using baby broccoli, or broccolini, because you can eat the whole thing, including the stem. Regular broccoli has a large stalk that is hard to digest for most people.

1 bunch baby broccoli, or broccolini

1 tablespoon coconut oil

2 teaspoons sea salt, divided

1 teaspoon freshly ground black pepper, divided

2 pounds boneless, skinless chicken breasts or thighs

2 tablespoons unsalted butter, divided

3 garlic cloves, peeled and minced

2 lemons; juice one and a half and slice the remaining half into (3 or 4) thin wheels

1 tablespoon capers

1 cup bone broth (homemade, page 78, or store-bought organic) or vegetable broth

2 tablespoons pine nuts

1. Preheat the oven to 450°F.
2. Arrange your clean baby broccoli on a baking sheet, keeping all the leaves. Drizzle with the coconut oil, 1 teaspoon of salt, and ½ teaspoon of pepper. Toss to coat well.
3. Roast for 20 minutes, or until the edges are lightly browning and slightly wilted. Do not overcook--they should still be vibrant green in color.
4. Pat your chicken dry with a paper towel, then sprinkle both sides with the remaining 1 teaspoon of salt and ½ teaspoon of pepper.
5. In a large skillet over medium-high heat, melt 1 tablespoon of butter, and add the garlic.
6. As the butter begins to brown, add half of the lemon juice and the chicken breasts, cooking for 3 minutes on each side. They should be golden brown and leaving brown bits on the pan surface. Set the chicken aside in a small baking dish.
7. Turn the heat to high, and the remaining tablespoon of butter, the rest of the lemon juice, and the capers to the pan. Sauté for 3 minutes, or until the capers start to pucker and wilt.
8. Pour in the bone broth, and use a spatula to scrape up the browned bits from the pan surface. Pour this sauce over the chicken in the baking dish.
9. Serve the chicken with the lemon wheels on top with a side of the baby broccoli, and sprinkle with the pine nuts.

> **CONTINUED ON NEXT PAGE**

Lemon Chicken and Roasted Baby Broccoli with Pine Nuts

> **CONTINUED**

Storage Note: The whole meal stores in airtight containers for 5 days. The chicken freezes well.

Recipe Tip: Make a dozen lemony chicken breasts and freeze for other meals. You can mix and match the chicken with a salad or a grain dish. Always have some handy in case you run out of options. Drop a container in a sink full of hot water to thaw in a pinch.

Per Serving Calories: 743; Total fat: 31g; Saturated fat: 14g; Sodium: 1,774mg; Carbohydrates: 7g; Fiber: 2g; Protein: 109g

Slow Cooker Mushroom and Onion Chicken

Serves 4 | Prep time: 15 minutes | Cook time: 5 hours | 5 Ingredients | DF | Paleo | Slow Cooker

Slow cooker meals are the best. It takes the fuss out of cooking. When mushrooms are cooked for long periods like this, not only do they impart an earthy richness to the dish, but their healing properties come out, adding beneficial fiber and loads of minerals.

2 pounds boneless, skinless chicken breasts

1 teaspoon sea salt, plus more for seasoning

½ teaspoon freshly ground black pepper, plus more for seasoning

2 tablespoons coconut oil

3 garlic cloves, peeled and minced

½ cup vegetable or bone broth, homemade (page 78) or store-bought organic

2 cups sliced mixed mushrooms (cremini, shiitake, button)

1 large sweet onion, sliced

1. Pat the chicken breasts dry, and season with salt and pepper.
2. In a large skillet over high heat, melt the coconut oil, and add the garlic. Sauté for 1 minute, until fragrant, then add your chicken breasts. Sear briefly until brown, about 2 minutes on each side.
3. Transfer the chicken to the slow cooker.
4. Add about half of the broth to the skillet, and use a spatula to deglaze the pan, scraping up the garlic and any brown bits, then pour into the slow cooker.
5. Add the mushrooms, onion, salt, pepper, and the rest of the broth to the slow cooker. Cook on Low for 5 hours and serve.

Storage Note: This dish can easily be made in large amounts and then frozen in individual servings for a go-to lunch or quick dinner.

Recipe Tip: You can add 2 tablespoons of cornstarch to the sauce at the end of cooking to thicken it if you'd like a more gravy-like consistency. You can also pre-sear the chicken and prepare the veggies and add them to the cooker in the morning before you leave for work so you'll have dinner waiting for you at night. How nice would that be?

Per Serving Calories: 330; Total fat: 10g; Saturated fat: 6g; Sodium: 717mg; Carbohydrates: 6g; Fiber: 1g; Protein: 54g

Mediterranean Slow-Cooked Chicken and Vegetables

Serves 4 | Prep time: 15 minutes | Cook time: 5 hours | DF | Paleo | Slow Cooker

You can't go wrong with a Mediterranean menu. Heart-healthy fats, gut-healthy vegetables, and flavorful fresh herbs make it great all around. I love using chicken thighs with the skin and bone for this recipe. It adds depth of flavor and more healthy fat, while the slow-cooked bones contribute many gut-healing minerals.

2 pounds bone-in chicken thighs

1 teaspoon sea salt, plus more for seasoning

½ teaspoon freshly ground black pepper, plus more for seasoning

2 tablespoons coconut oil

3 garlic cloves, peeled and minced

1 teaspoon finely chopped fresh rosemary

½ teaspoon finely chopped fresh thyme

½ cup bone or vegetable broth, divided

1 large green bell pepper, cored and sliced into long strips

1 large red bell pepper, cored and sliced into long strips

1 large yellow bell pepper, cored and sliced into long strips

1 green zucchini, sliced into wheels

1 large sweet onion, sliced

1. Pat the chicken thighs dry, and season with salt and pepper.

2. In a large skillet over high heat, melt the coconut oil. Add the garlic and sauté for 1 minute, until fragrant, then add the chicken thighs. Sear just enough to brown each side, about 2 minutes per side. Transfer to the slow cooker. Add the salt, pepper, rosemary, thyme, and most of the broth, reserving a couple of tablespoons for the next step.

3. Add about 2 tablespoons of broth to the skillet, and use a spatula to deglaze the pan, scraping up the garlic and any brown bits, then pour into the slow cooker. Cook on Low for 3 hours.

4. After 3 hours, add the bell peppers, zucchini, and onion to the slow cooker. Cook for a final 2 hours on Low and serve.

Storage Note: This dish stores, refrigerated, in an airtight container for up to 5 days. It also freezes well.

Recipe Tip: Adding the vegetables halfway through the cooking process helps keep them from getting too soft, but it's not necessary if adding them earlier will reduce your time and fuss.

Per Serving Calories: 601; Total fat: 41g; Saturated fat: 16g; Sodium: 738mg; Carbohydrates: 14g; Fiber: 2g; Protein: 43g

Chicken, Green Chile, Corn & Millet Casserole

Serves 4 | Prep time: 10 minutes | Cook time: 1 hour 10 minutes | Quick Prep

One of the tough things about going gluten-free is that we crave that grounding, filling quality that comes with bread or pasta. If you have such a craving, this casserole will satisfy your desire in short order—without the inflammatory qualities of gluten-filled products.

2 pounds boneless, skinless chicken thighs

1 teaspoon sea salt

½ teaspoon freshly ground black pepper

2 tablespoons coconut oil or ghee, divided

2 garlic cloves, peeled and minced

1 (8-ounce) can green chile peppers, mild heat, chopped small

1 large red bell pepper, cored and diced

1 large sweet onion, diced

1 (16-ounce) can sweet corn or 1 (16-ounce) bag frozen corn

1½ cups millet, rinsed

6 cups vegetable or bone broth, homemade (page 78) or store-bought organic

1. Preheat the oven to 350°F.
2. Pat the chicken thighs dry, and season with salt and pepper.
3. In a large stockpot over medium-high heat, melt 1 tablespoon of coconut oil, and add the garlic. Sauté for 1 minute, until fragrant, then add the chicken thighs. Cook for 3 minutes on each side, until cooked through. Set aside to cool.
4. Add the remaining 1 tablespoon of coconut oil to the pot, add the chiles, bell pepper, onion, corn, salt, and pepper, and sauté for 3 minutes, until the onion is translucent.
5. Add the millet and broth, and bring to a boil, then lower the heat to a simmer and cook, covered, for 30 minutes.
6. When the chicken is cool, place on a cutting board and chop into bite-size pieces.
7. In a medium casserole dish, combine the millet mixture and chicken. Mix until incorporated well.
8. Transfer to the oven and bake for 30 minutes and serve.

Storage Note: This dish stores well refrigerated in an airtight container for up to 5 days. It also freezes well.

Recipe Tip: This is an easy recipe to make vegan—just omit the chicken and use veggie broth. Try adding a Mexican spice blend to the millet before cooking for more Southwestern flavor.

Per Serving Calories: 757; Total fat: 20g; Saturated fat: 9g; Sodium: 1,270mg; Carbohydrates: 86g; Fiber: 11g; Protein: 61g

Chinese Garlic Chicken Stir-Fry

Serves 4 | Prep time: 15 minutes, plus at least 1 hour to marinate | Cook time: 20 minutes | DF | NF

Too much restaurant food is filled with preservatives like MSG and unhealthy fats, which are terrible for the gut. But ordering takeout Chinese is so fun. Here's a gut-friendly substitute you can enjoy guilt-free.

FOR THE MARINADE

1 tablespoon grated fresh ginger root

1 tablespoon toasted sesame oil

2 tablespoons apple cider vinegar (I use Bragg's)

½ cup tamari

2 garlic cloves, peeled and minced

FOR THE STIR-FRY

2 pounds boneless, skinless chicken thighs, cut into chunks

2 tablespoons toasted sesame oil, divided

2 garlic cloves, peeled and minced

1 onion, sliced

1 carrot, peeled and sliced into discs

1 cup cremini and button mushrooms, sliced

1 cup broccoli florets

1 red bell pepper, cored and sliced

1 cup snow peas

½ tablespoon Gomashio (page 172)

TO MAKE THE MARINADE

In a small bowl, combine the ginger, sesame oil, vinegar, tamari, and garlic, and whisk well.

TO MAKE THE STIR-FRY

1. Combine the chicken and marinade in a zip-top bag, and place it in the fridge for at least 1 hour, or overnight.
2. In a large skillet over medium-high heat, heat 1 tablespoon of sesame oil. Add the garlic and onion, and sauté until the onion is translucent, 3 to 4 minutes.
3. Add the carrot, mushrooms, broccoli, bell pepper, and snow peas to the pan, and sauté for another 5 minutes, until tender. Transfer to a plate and set aside.
4. Heat the remaining 1 tablespoon of sesame oil, and add the chicken to the pan. Cook for about 3 minutes on each side, until cooked through, returning the vegetables to the pan at the end to heat through.
5. Sprinkle with the Gomashio and serve.

Storage Note: This dish stores well refrigerated in an airtight container for up to 5 days.

Recipe Tip: This is an easy recipe to flip to vegan. Just omit the chicken. Served over wild rice, this is a nice treat.

Per Serving Calories: 438; Total fat: 20g; Saturated fat: 4g; Sodium: 2,235mg; Carbohydrates: 15g; Fiber: 4g; Protein: 51g

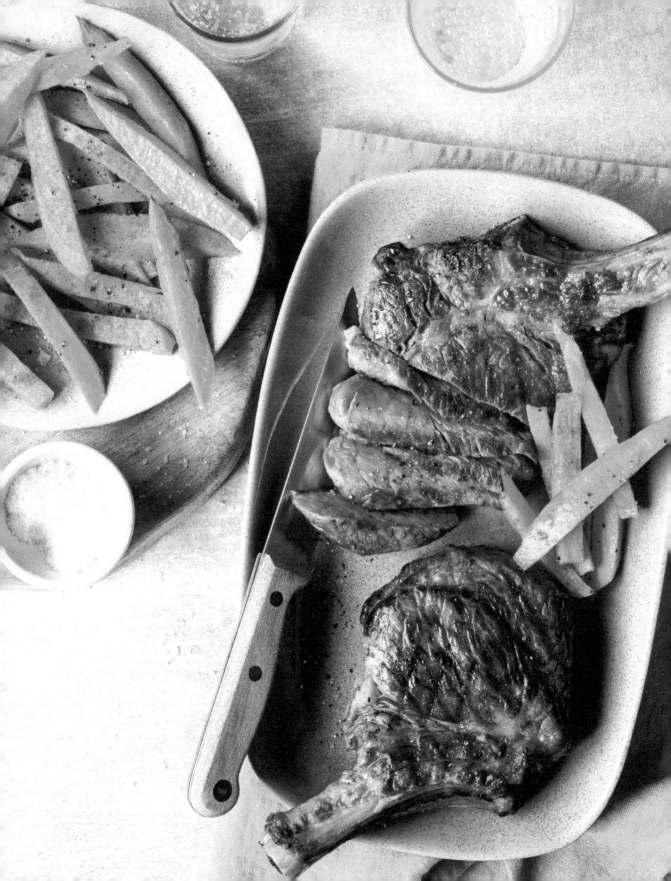

Beef, Pork, and Lamb

Opposite: Cast-Iron Rib Eyes with Sweet Potato Fries, page 126

Slow Cooker Beef Bourguignon

Serves 4 | Prep time: 20 minutes | Cook time: 6 to 8 hours | DF | Slow Cooker

Here we have one of my all-time favorite classic dishes. This rich, deep, comforting meal is incredibly satiating and will leave you content. The original recipe calls for ingredients that can cause some belly distress, so I've modified the classic for a more gut-friendly experience.

2 tablespoons coconut oil

2 pounds beef stew meat

1 onion, diced

1 pound carrots, peeled and cut into bite-size discs

1 pound baby round potatoes, if you can find them; otherwise, baby reds quartered

2 dried bay leaves

4 garlic cloves, peeled and minced

1 cup frozen pearl onions

8 to 10 cremini mushrooms, halved

2 cups bone broth (homemade, page 78, or store-bought organic)

2 cups Burgundy red wine (Cabernet will do)

1 teaspoon sea salt

1 teaspoon freshly ground black pepper

1. In a large skillet over medium-high heat, melt the coconut oil. Sauté the beef until browned on all sides, about 6 minutes.

2. Place the onion, carrots, and potatoes on the bottom of the slow cooker, then add the beef with the drippings from the pan. Add the bay leaves, garlic, pearl onions, mushrooms, broth, wine, salt, and pepper on top. Cook on Low for 6 hours.

3. At 6 hours, check to see if the beef is tender; the chunks should fall apart when pressed with a fork. If not, cook for 2 more hours. Remove the bay leaves before serving.

Storage Note: This stew will keep, refrigerated and covered with a lid, for 4 to 5 days. You can also freeze this meal; it makes a great grab-and-go lunch.

Recipe Tip: You can add a couple of tablespoons of potato starch or cornstarch near the end, around hour 5, to thicken the stew into more of a gravy-like consistency.

Per Serving Calories: 538; Total fat: 19g; Saturated fat: 10g; Sodium: 688mg; Carbohydrates: 36g; Fiber: 7g; Protein: 55g

Slow Cooker Paleo Chili

Serves 4 | Prep time: 20 minutes | Cook time: 6 hours | DF | Paleo | Slow Cooker

My mom says everyone should be good at cooking chili. That's because it's a good fallback recipe when you're out of ideas. Everyone loves a warm bowl of chili—it's delicious and hearty, and this one won't destroy your gut with hard-to-digest ingredients.

1 tablespoon coconut oil

1 pound grass-fed ground beef

1 green bell pepper, cored and diced

1 red bell pepper, cored and diced

1 onion, diced

2 cups bone broth (homemade, page 78, or store-bought organic)

4 garlic cloves, peeled and minced

1 tablespoon paprika

1 tablespoon ground cumin

½ teaspoon chipotle chili powder

1 teaspoon sea salt

1 teaspoon freshly ground black pepper

1 cup chopped fresh cilantro, for topping

1 small ripe avocado, sliced, for topping

1. In a large skillet over high heat, melt the coconut oil. Add the ground beef and cook, stirring, until well browned, 3 to 4 minutes.
2. Transfer the meat to your slow cooker along with the green and red bell peppers, onion, broth, garlic, paprika, cumin, chipotle powder, salt, and pepper. Stir to combine.
3. Cook on Low for 6 hours.
4. Serve topped with the cilantro and avocado slices.

Storage Note: This will keep, refrigerated and covered, for 4 days. You can also freeze this meal for easy lunches and dinners when you're on the run.

Recipe Tip: This chili can be a main course or a side. Plus, it can be added to many other recipes. Try it over quinoa or with a lean chicken breast, or use it to top mixed greens for a Tex-Mex salad. Top with a fried egg for a filling, delicious breakfast.

Per Serving Calories: 337; Total fat: 22g; Saturated fat: 8g; Sodium: 554mg; Carbohydrates: 11g; Fiber: 5g; Protein: 25g

Cast-Iron Rib Eyes with Sweet Potato Fries

Serves 2 | Prep time: 10 minutes, plus at least 30 minutes to rest | Cook time: 45 minutes | 5 Ingredients | DF | Paleo

I have a lot of different recipes vying for my favorite go-to meal, but this one never leaves the top 5. I love a juicy, medium-rare steak, and I prefer rib eyes with the bone. Meat cooked on the bone imparts more flavor and nutrients—and nothing complements it better than some form of potato. I used to love French fries until I realized how bad the deep-fried fat was for the gut. Once you discover these sweet potato fries, you will never look back.

2 (1-pound) bone-in rib eye steaks

1½ tablespoons plus 1 teaspoon coconut oil, divided

1 teaspoon sea salt, plus more for seasoning

1 teaspoon freshly ground black pepper, plus more for seasoning

4 large garnet sweet potatoes, peeled and sliced into skinny, fingerlike wedges

1 teaspoon paprika

1 teaspoon garlic salt

1. To prep the steaks, cover them in ½ tablespoon of coconut oil, season with salt and pepper, then allow to sit at room temperature for at least 30 minutes before cooking.

2. Preheat the oven to 420°F.

3. On a large baking sheet, toss the sweet potato fries in 1 teaspoon of coconut oil to coat thoroughly, then spread in an even layer across the sheet.

4. Sprinkle liberally with the salt, pepper, paprika, and garlic salt.

5. Roast for 30 minutes. Remove from the oven, turn the fries over with a spatula, then return to the oven for another 10 to 15 minutes, or until browning at the edges and tender.

6. Meanwhile, heat a large cast-iron skillet over medium-high heat. Heat the remaining 1 tablespoon of coconut oil until it pools and glistens. You can splash a few drops of water on the pan to see if it's hot enough—it will spatter when it's ready.

7. Place the steaks in the skillet, and cook about 3 to 4 minutes on each side for medium-rare.

8. Transfer the steaks to a cutting board and cover with foil, allowing them to rest for 7 minutes.

9. Slice the steak into strips. I love serving the steak on the cutting board and the fries in a metal mixing bowl lined with a piece of newspaper. It's rustic and fun.

Storage Note: Steak will keep, refrigerated and covered in an air-tight container, for 4 to 5 days.

Recipe Tip: Marinating the steaks in olive oil, sea salt, pepper, and garlic salt for a few hours before cooking will tenderize the meat even more. Be prepared for a smoky kitchen when cooking meat on a cast-iron skillet at a high temperature. If you like a crispier fry on your potatoes, you can cook for longer than 40 minutes. Do not crowd the sweet potatoes, because they will not get firm or crunchy.

Per Serving Calories: 1,472; Total fat: 110g; Saturated fat: 51g; Sodium: 1,148mg; Carbohydrates: 58g; Fiber: 9g; Protein: 57g

Grass-Fed Bison Quinoa Bowl with Turmeric-Ginger Sauce

Serves 2 | Prep time: 10 minutes | Cook time: 10 minutes 5 | Ingredients | DF | Quick Prep

This is another easy-peasy go-to meal that makes for quick lunches and dinners and, yes, even breakfast. The tangy Turmeric-Ginger Sauce is not only delicious, brightening up this otherwise bland dish, but it also has anti-inflammatory properties to soothe and heal your belly.

1 tablespoon coconut oil

2 garlic cloves, peeled and minced

2 pounds grass-fed ground bison

4 cups cooked quinoa

1 cup Turmeric-Ginger Sauce (page 98)

1. In a large skillet over medium-high heat, melt the coconut oil. Add the garlic and sauté for 1 to 2 minutes, until fragrant.
2. Add the ground bison, and stir until it has browned and cooked through, about 5 minutes.
3. Divide the quinoa between 2 bowls, and top each with half of the ground bison.
4. Top each portion of bison and quinoa with a half cup of Turmeric-Ginger Sauce before serving.

Storage Note: The bison and quinoa mixture will keep, refrigerated and covered with a lid, for 4 to 5 days. You can also freeze this meal and thaw a container for an easy lunch.

Recipe Tip: The trick to keeping this meal so simple is pre-making your dressing and quinoa. Always store the dressing in a small container on the side of the meal and add before eating. This dressing is good cold or warmed up.

Per Serving Calories: 1,299; Total fat: 59g; Saturated fat: 22g; Sodium: 403mg; Carbohydrates: 94g; Fiber: 14g; Protein: 116g

Slow Cooker Swedish Meatballs and Mushroom Sauce

Serves 4 | Prep time: 15 minutes | Cook time: 4 hours 10 minutes | Slow Cooker

Comfort food score: 10 out of 10! This recipe is creamy, rich, and rustic. I always feel a bit guilty eating it because it has a decadent quality, but have no fear. It's a gut-friendly, guilt-free crowd-pleaser.

½ cup gluten-free bread crumbs (I like Ian's)

2 tablespoons ghee or melted coconut oil, divided

1 small onion, minced

2 teaspoons sea salt, divided, plus more for seasoning

½ teaspoon freshly ground black pepper, plus more for seasoning

1 pound lean, grass-fed ground beef

1 pound lean ground pork

1 large egg

1¼ cup bone broth (homemade, page 78, or store-bought organic)

2 cups cremini mushrooms, chopped

¼ cup plain Greek yogurt

1. In a large dry skillet over medium heat, toast the bread crumbs for 2 to 3 minutes, until lightly browned and crisp. Transfer to a small mixing bowl.

2. In the same skillet over medium heat, melt 1 tablespoon of ghee, and add the onion and salt and pepper to taste. Sauté until translucent, 3 to 4 minutes

3. In a large mixing bowl, combine the beef, pork, 1 teaspoon of salt, pepper, egg, sautéed onion, and bread crumbs. Mix well, and make golf ball–size meatballs, setting aside on a plate.

4. In the same skillet over high heat, melt another tablespoon of ghee.

5. Add the meatballs to the skillet and brown quickly, about 1 to 2 minutes total, and transfer to the slow cooker.

6. Pour ¼ cup of broth into the skillet, and deglaze the pan, scraping the browned bits off the bottom, then pour into the slow cooker.

7. Add the chopped mushrooms, yogurt, the remaining 1 cup of bone broth, and the remaining teaspoon of salt to the slow cooker.

8. Cover, cook on Low for 4 hours, and serve.

Storage Note: You can make the meatballs ahead of time and refrigerate for up to 5 days; you can also freeze them.

Recipe Tip: If you are dairy sensitive, you can omit the yogurt, though the sauce will be less thick and creamy. If desired, you can add 2 tablespoons of potato starch toward the end, around hour 3, to thicken the juices.

Per Serving Calories: 649; Total fat: 39g; Saturated fat: 11g; Sodium: 1,166mg; Carbohydrates: 23g; Fiber: 3g; Protein: 48g

Slow Cooker Kalua Pork & Cabbage

Serves 8 | Prep time: 15 minutes | Cook time: 16 hours | 5 Ingredients | DF | NF | Paleo | Slow Cooker

I was introduced to this Hawaiian staple by a dear friend. It's easy and succulent, and everyone will think you were in the kitchen for days slaving over a hot oven. Nothing could be further from the truth. Slow-cooked bone-in meat is a densely nutritious and easy-to-digest food. This dish is laden with minerals and flavor, and the cabbage is rich in vitamins K and C. It's good for more than dinner, too! Try serving at breakfast with a soft-boiled egg, for lunch in a lettuce and flatbread wrap, and in a small to-go cup as a quick snack.

1 (5-pound) bone-in
   pork butt roast

1½ tablespoons sea salt

5 garlic cloves, peeled
   and crushed

1 small head green cabbage
   (about 2 pounds)

1. Salt the pork well, covering it liberally and thoroughly.
2. Place the pork and the crushed garlic cloves in a slow cooker. Cook on Low for 16 hours. Do not add any liquid.
3. Once the roast is tender and falling apart, transfer to a large plate. Shred the meat with 2 forks. Set aside.
4. Shred the cabbage using a large chef's knife or a food processor.
5. Place a large skillet over medium heat. Add a few tablespoons of the pork juices from the slow cooker, stir in the cabbage, and cook until tender, 3 to 5 minutes.
6. Taste the juices in the slow cooker for salt levels. If they're too salty for your taste, reserve in mason jars to use for cooking grains or beans.
7. Place the shredded pork back into the slow cooker to coat with the juices, and serve with the cabbage.

Storage Note: This dish will keep refrigerated for 1 week in an airtight container. Make this on a Sunday and have meals for the whole week. Store in individual containers in the freezer.

Recipe Tip: I also like to serve this dish with a cup of fermented vegetables like sauerkraut. See the recipe for Dill and Caraway Sauerkraut on page 167 to make your own.

Per Serving Calories: 550; Total fat: 35g; Saturated fat: 13g; Sodium: 1,501mg; Carbohydrates: 6g; Fiber: 2g; Protein: 51g

Slow Cooker Posole Pork Stew

Serves 4 | Prep time: 20 minutes | Cook time: 6 to 8 hours | Slow Cooker

This Mexican favorite traditionally takes days to prepare and is often only served for the holidays. This slow cooker version takes out all the fuss. The result is a tangy, rich, meaty bowl of stew that everyone will love . . . including your gut. The broth is rich in minerals and gut-healthy nutrients.

FOR THE STEW

1 (3- to 4-pound) pork butt, bone-in

1 tablespoon ghee or melted coconut oil

1 tablespoon sea salt

1 (15.5-ounce) can hominy, drained (you can find this in the ethnic section of almost any grocer or online)

1 dried bay leaf

4 garlic cloves, peeled and minced

1 onion, diced

2 carrots, peeled and diced

1 dried red chile (optional)

1 teaspoon red chili powder

1 teaspoon freshly ground black pepper

FOR TOPPING (OPTIONAL)

Shredded green cabbage

Chopped fresh cilantro

Dried oregano

Sliced lime wedges

1. Coat the pork butt with the ghee, rub down with salt in all the nooks and crannies, and transfer to the slow cooker.
2. Add the hominy, bay leaf, garlic, onion, carrots, chile, chili powder, and pepper to the slow cooker.
3. Cook on Low for 6 hours, or until tender.
4. Transfer the pork to a cutting board, and shred with 2 forks. Return to the slow cooker, and stir to combine.
5. Remove the bay leaf. Serve each portion in a big soup bowl, and arrange the toppings (if using) in small bowls to be added at the table.

Storage Note: This stew will keep, refrigerated and covered with a lid, for 4 to 5 days. You can also freeze this stew for quick meals during the week. Keep toppings separate, and add just before eating.

Recipe Tip: The dried chile pod is an authentic ingredient that adds gorgeous color and flavor. If you can find one, it's a wonderful addition, but not necessary.

Per Serving Calories: 663; Total fat: 39g; Saturated fat: 15g; Sodium: 903mg; Carbohydrates: 23g; Fiber: 5g; Protein: 53g

Quinoa Kibbeh with Lentils and Laban

Serves 4 | Prep time: 20 minutes | Cook time: 20 minutes

Kibbeh is an ancient recipe, and there are many versions. This one is easy and, of course, gut-friendly.

2 cups green lentils, rinsed

3 cups bone broth (homemade, page 78, or store-bought organic)

2 teaspoons sea salt, divided

2 pounds ground lamb, grass-fed

3 cups cooked quinoa

1 teaspoon freshly ground black pepper

¼ teaspoon ground cumin

1 teaspoon ground allspice

2 medium onions, minced

¼ cup pine nuts

2 tablespoons coconut oil or ghee

1 cup Cucumber Laban (page 171)

1. Preheat the oven to 375°F, and place a cast-iron skillet in the oven to heat.
2. In a medium saucepan, cover the lentils with the broth, add 1 teaspoon of salt, and bring to a low boil for 20 minutes, or until the liquid has evaporated and the lentils are tender. Cover and set aside.
3. Meanwhile, in a large mixing bowl, combine the lamb, quinoa, the remaining 1 teaspoon of salt, pepper, cumin, allspice, onions, and pine nuts.
4. Form the mixture into balls about the size of a large egg.
5. Using a potholder or two, carefully take the cast-iron skillet out of the oven and add the coconut oil.
6. Place your kibbeh balls in the skillet and return to the oven, again using a potholder.
7. Cook for 20 minutes, until lightly browned.
8. Serve the kibbeh balls with a side of lentils and Cucumber Laban.

Storage Note: The kibbeh keep, refrigerated in an airtight container, for 4 to 5 days. You can also freeze this meal for easy lunches later.

Recipe Tip: I like to turn my broiler on when the kibbeh have cooked for 15 minutes so that they can brown for the last 5 minutes.

Per Serving Calories: 1,187; Total fat: 48g; Saturated fat: 19g; Sodium: 1,257mg; Carbohydrates: 104g; Fiber: 66g; Protein: 85g

Moroccan Lamb Tagine

Serves 4 | Prep time: 20 minutes | Cook time: 1 hour 40 minutes | Paleo

This fragrant, succulent dish is commonly served in a gorgeous Moroccan clay tagine pot. It's a dish that is sure to impress, especially if you can find a tagine pot to serve it in. The combinations of spices can help soothe the gut, but if you have issues digesting beans, you may wish to omit the chickpeas.

2 teaspoons coconut oil or ghee, divided

2 pounds lamb stew meat

1 large onion, roughly chopped

3 garlic cloves, peeled and minced

2 teaspoons grated fresh ginger root

1 teaspoon ground cumin

½ teaspoon ground coriander

½ teaspoon paprika

1 teaspoon sea salt

1 teaspoon freshly ground black pepper

2 cups bone broth (homemade, page 78, or store-bought organic)

1 (16-ounce) can chickpeas, drained

1 medium butternut squash, peeled, seeded, and chopped into cubes

2 tablespoons minced fresh mint

1. In a large skillet over medium-high heat, melt 1 teaspoon of coconut oil. Add the lamb meat, and cook until browned, 4 to 5 minutes. Set aside.

2. Lower the heat to medium, and add the remaining teaspoon of coconut oil and the onion, garlic, ginger, cumin, coriander, paprika, salt, and pepper. Sauté until a very fragrant paste forms, 1 to 2 minutes.

3. Add the broth, and deglaze the pan, stirring up whatever has stuck to the bottom of the skillet, then add back the lamb, cover, and lower the heat to medium-low.

4. Cook for about 1 hour, or until the meat is tender.

5. Add the chickpeas and butternut squash. Cook for another 30 minutes, or until you can pierce the squash easily with a knife.

6. Sprinkle with the minced mint and serve.

Storage Note: This dish will keep, refrigerated and covered with a lid, for 4 to 5 days. This also freezes well for quick meals on the go.

Recipe Tip: There is a spice blend called *ras el hanout* that can make dishes like this a lot easier to flavor without having to buy each spice individually. It usually includes coriander, paprika, ginger, cumin, clove, and cinnamon or different variations of similar spices. It's a great addition to any spice rack. This dish can easily be made deliciously vegetarian: Just omit the lamb, add more vegetables of your choice, and substitute vegetable broth for the bone broth.

Per Serving Calories: 541; Total fat: 16g; Saturated fat: 7g; Sodium: 960mg; Carbohydrates: 45g; Fiber: 9g; Protein: 53g

Feta Lamb Burgers with Rosemary Baby Reds

Serves 4 | Prep time: 20 minutes | Cook time: 40 minutes

This salty, rich, hearty Irish dish is a classic. And the basic ingredients keep it both gut-friendly and easy to whip up.

5 small baby red potatoes, quartered

2 tablespoons coconut oil or ghee, divided

2 teaspoons sea salt, divided

1 teaspoon freshly ground black pepper, divided

1 teaspoon paprika

1 tablespoon minced fresh rosemary

2 pounds ground lamb

½ cup feta cheese, plus 1 tablespoon crumbled, divided

½ cup chopped fresh parsley

½ teaspoon dried oregano

1. Preheat the oven to 425°F.
2. Place the baby red potatoes on a large baking sheet, and coat with 1 tablespoon of the coconut oil, then sprinkle liberally with 1 teaspoon of salt, ½ teaspoon of pepper, and the paprika and rosemary.
3. Roast for 35 to 40 minutes, or until nicely browned.
4. Meanwhile, in a large mixing bowl, combine the lamb, ½ cup of feta cheese, the parsley and oregano, and the remaining 1 teaspoon of salt and ½ teaspoon of pepper. Mix well.
5. Form the lamb mixture into 4 palm-size patties.
6. In a large skillet over medium heat, melt the remaining tablespoon of coconut oil. Add the lamb patties, cooking 2 at a time, depending on the size of your skillet—be sure not to crowd the pan. Cook for about 2 to 3 minutes per side for medium-rare burgers.
7. Sprinkle with the remaining tablespoon of crumbled feta, and serve with the potatoes.

Storage Note: These burgers keep, refrigerated and covered with a lid, for 4 to 5 days. You can also freeze this meal. It keeps very well and is a good "grab and go" option for lunches.

Recipe Tip: I like to use a cast-iron skillet for lamb; it seems to impart more flavor. I also like to throw the potatoes into the skillet on high heat at the end of roasting with a teaspoon of ghee to give them a quick sauté. This also adds flavor.

Per Serving Calories: 855; Total fat: 65g; Saturated fat: 33g; Sodium: 1,288mg; Carbohydrates: 25g; Fiber: 4g; Protein: 44g

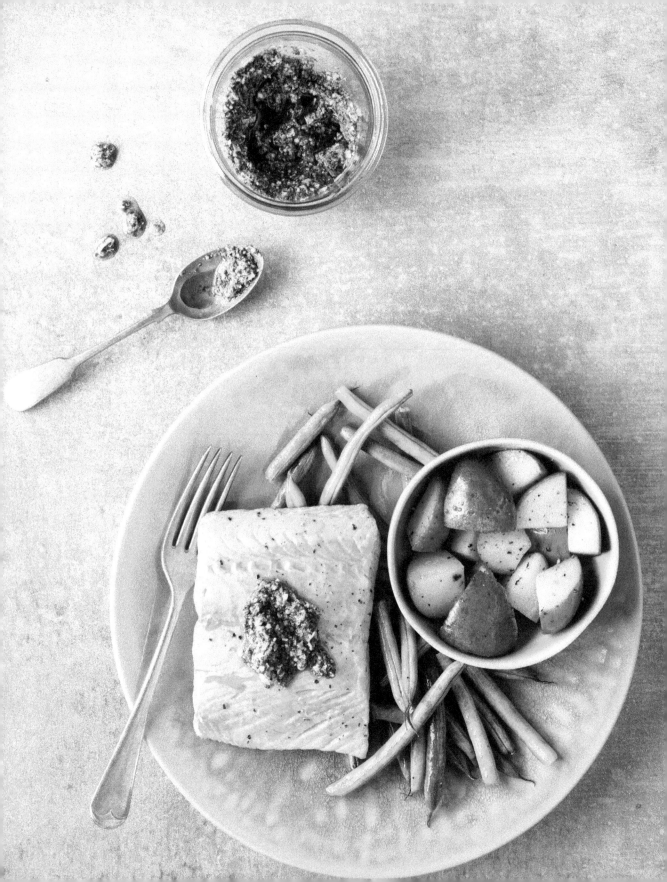

Fish and Seafood

Opposite: Pesto Salmon, Green Beans, and Baby Reds, page 145

Prosciutto-Wrapped Cod on Forbidden Rice

Serves 4 | Prep time: 5 minutes | Cook time: 10 minutes | 5 Ingredients | Quick Prep | NF | Paleo

This is such an easy recipe to make. Plus, the simple ingredients are both easy to digest and bursting with flavor.

4 skinless cod fillets (about 2 pounds), at room temperature

8 slices prosciutto

2 tablespoons ghee

1 garlic clove, peeled and minced

2 cups forbidden rice, cooked

Squeeze of lemon juice

Sea salt, if desired, (prosciutto is quite salty already)

1. Pat the cod fillets dry with a paper towel.
2. On a cutting board or dry countertop, lay out your prosciutto in vertical strips, 2 per piece of cod.
3. Place the cod across the strips horizontally, then fold the prosciutto across the cod like swaddling a baby in a blanket. Keep it snug, but not too tight.
4. In a large skillet over medium heat, melt the ghee. Add the garlic and prosciutto-wrapped fillets, and cook for about 4 to 5 minutes on each side. The edges of the prosciutto should begin to brown and curl up, and the fish should be firm but still tender.
5. Serve immediately on top of a bowl of warm forbidden rice with a squeeze of lemon juice and a sprinkle of salt, if necessary.

Storage Note: This dish will keep, refrigerated and covered with a lid, for 3 days.

Recipe Tip: For a more filling meal, you can add some sautéed spinach and sprinkle with slivered almonds.

Per Serving Calories: 357; Total fat: 13g; Saturated fat: 6g; Sodium: 800mg; Carbohydrates: 11g; Fiber: 1g; Protein: 50g

Baked Cod with Spinach and Capers

Serves 4 | Prep time: 5 minutes | Cook time: 15 minutes | NF | Quick Prep

Flaky, lemony, healthy, and gut-friendly—what a great dish. Cod is filled with healthy fats, which your gut loves, and the combination of spices, garlic, and lemon make this dish a taste bud favorite. The lemon and caper spinach side adds more delicious nutrients and is a breeze to digest.

FOR THE COD

4 skinless cod fillets (about 2 pounds), at room temperature

5 tablespoons ghee, divided

¼ cup freshly squeezed lemon juice

⅓ cup gluten-free all-purpose flour (I like King Arthur)

1 teaspoon sea salt

¼ teaspoon freshly ground black pepper

½ teaspoon paprika or Aleppo pepper

5 garlic cloves, peeled and minced

FOR THE SPINACH

1 tablespoon ghee

3 garlic cloves, peeled and minced

2 tablespoons capers

1 tablespoon freshly squeezed lemon juice

1 (16-ounce) bag fresh, baby spinach

½ teaspoon sea salt

¼ teaspoon freshly ground black pepper

TO MAKE THE COD

1. Preheat the oven to 400°F.
2. Pat the cod fillets dry with a paper towel.
3. Melt 4 tablespoons of ghee in a small saucepan, and pour into a small dish. Add the lemon juice, mix well, and set aside.
4. In a medium mixing bowl, mix the flour, salt, pepper, and paprika. Set aside.
5. In a large skillet over medium-high heat, heat the remaining 1 tablespoon of ghee.
6. Dip one piece of cod into the lemon ghee dish, then into the flour bowl.
7. Place the coated cod in the hot skillet, and sear for 1 minute on each side. Set aside.
8. Place your coated, seared fillets in a baking dish. Pour over the remaining lemon ghee, and add the garlic.
9. Bake for 8 to 10 minutes, or until the fish is flaky and tender.

TO MAKE THE SPINACH

1. Meanwhile, in a large skillet over medium-high heat, melt 1 tablespoon of ghee.
2. Add the garlic and capers and sauté, stirring continuously so the garlic does not burn, until the capers begin to pucker or dimple, about 3 minutes.
3. Add the lemon juice, and sauté for another minute or so before adding the spinach. Cook the spinach until it wilts down, then add the salt and pepper. Remove from the heat and arrange on a plate.
4. Serve the cooked cod on top of the bed of spinach.

> **CONTINUED ON NEXT PAGE**

Baked Cod with Spinach and Capers

> **CONTINUED**

Storage Note: The fish will keep, refrigerated and covered with a lid, for 3 days. The fish also freezes well.

Recipe Tip: The spinach is best eaten immediately, but you can save the fish as leftovers and add it to a salad for lunch or dinner. It's even yummy cold.

Per Serving Calories: 422; Total fat: 22g; Saturated fat: 12g; Sodium: 1,084mg; Carbohydrates: 14g; Fiber: 4g; Protein: 44g

Zoodles with Lemon-Garlic Shrimp

Serves 4 | Prep time: 10 minutes | Cook time: 5 minutes | Paleo | Quick Prep

My husband is a major pasta fan, so you can imagine his distress when I put him on a gut-healthy diet and *no* pasta was on the menu. He said zucchini noodles were a sin—until I made him this dish. Lemony, juicy shrimp with garlicky zucchini noodles in a wine sauce: You can't go wrong.

4 large zucchini

2 tablespoons coconut oil or ghee, divided

4 garlic cloves, peeled and minced, divided

1 pound raw shrimp, peeled, deveined, and rinsed

1 lemon, zested for 1 teaspoon of zest, then juiced

1 teaspoon sea salt

1 teaspoon freshly ground black pepper

Pinch red pepper flakes

¼ cup white wine or chicken or vegetable broth

¼ cup chopped fresh parsley

1. Spiralize the zucchini or peel into thin strips with a veggie peeler. Set aside.
2. In a large skillet over medium-high heat, melt 1 tablespoon of coconut oil, and sauté half the garlic for 30 seconds, or until fragrant, then add the shrimp. Cook for 1 minute on each side, until pink and opaque, then transfer to a plate.
3. In the same skillet, melt another tablespoon of coconut oil, and sauté the remaining garlic for 30 seconds before adding the lemon zest and juice, salt, pepper, and red pepper flakes. Stir well.
4. Add the wine and deglaze the pan, scraping the bottom to release any delicious bits of flavor.
5. Add the zoodles for just long enough to heat up them up and coat them with the sauce, no more than 2 minutes.
6. Add the shrimp back in, and toss to combine.
7. Sprinkle with the chopped parsley and serve.

Storage Note: This dish will keep, refrigerated in an airtight container, for 2 to 3 days.

Recipe Tip: When heating this dish up, I like to throw in about ¼ cup of bone or veggie broth to reconstitute the lemon-garlic sauce.

Per Serving Calories: 245; Total fat: 9g; Saturated fat: 6g; Sodium: 290mg; Carbohydrates: 14g; Fiber: 4g; Protein: 28g

Halibut Fish Taco Bowl with Lemon-Cilantro Cream Sauce

Serves 2 | Prep time: 20 minutes | Cook time: 10 minutes

For me, nothing says summer like fish tacos. It's hard to find a white fish as flaky and juicy as halibut. It stands on its own, but when coupled with this lemony, fragrant cilantro sauce, it's to die for. The gut is not crazy about corn, and certainly not flour, so creating this taco bowl without tortillas was important—but so was making sure taco lovers didn't miss out.

FOR THE BOWL

2 thick pieces halibut (about 1 pound total)

1 tablespoon coconut oil or ghee

2 garlic cloves, peeled and minced

Sea salt

Freshly ground black pepper

2 cups wild rice, cooked

FOR THE LEMON-CILANTRO CREAM SAUCE

1 bunch fresh cilantro, roughly chopped

1 garlic clove, peeled and minced

¼ cup plain Greek yogurt

¼ cup water, plus more if needed

2 tablespoons freshly squeezed lemon juice

1 teaspoon sea salt

½ teaspoon freshly ground black pepper

FOR THE TOPPINGS

½ cup green cabbage, finely shredded (I use a cheese grater to get it fine)

½ cup red radish, finely shredded

2 teaspoons apple cider vinegar (I use Bragg's)

Sea salt

Freshly ground black pepper

TO MAKE THE LEMON-CILANTRO CREAM SAUCE

In a blender, combine the cilantro, garlic, yogurt, water, lemon juice, salt, and pepper, and blend until smooth. Add more water by tablespoons if necessary to reach a very smooth consistency. Set aside in a small bowl.

TO MAKE THE TOPPINGS

In a small mixing bowl, combine cabbage, radish, vinegar, salt, and pepper. Mix well. Set aside.

TO MAKE THE BOWL

1. Pat the halibut dry with a paper towel. Set aside and allow to come to room temperature.
2. In a large skillet over medium-high heat, melt the coconut oil. Add the garlic, and sauté for 1 minute, being careful not to burn it.
3. Add the halibut and cook for 3 minutes on each side, or until tender and flaky with the edges browning a bit.
4. Divide the rice between two bowls. Top with the halibut, and drizzle with the lemon-cilantro cream sauce. Top with the shredded radish and cabbage toppings, season with salt and pepper, and serve.

Storage Note: This dish will keep, refrigerated and covered in an airtight container, for 3 to 4 days. You can also freeze this meal for quick lunches. Keep the dressing and topping separate when storing.

Recipe Tip: If you want to omit the dairy, you can use plain coconut yogurt instead. If you prefer a spicy kick to the sauce, you can add ¼ teaspoon of ground cayenne when blending the ingredients.

Per Serving Calories: 558; Total fat: 13g; Saturated fat: 6g; Sodium: 1,132mg; Carbohydrates: 40g; Fiber: 4g; Protein: 71g

Spinach Fish Bake

Serves 4 | Prep time: 15 minutes | Cook time: 1 hour | NF

This Spinach Fish Bake is a hearty, juicy, and delicious dish that everyone loves. It is nutritionally dense, with so many veggies and luscious pieces of tender, easy-to-digest fish.

2½ pounds firm white fish (such as cod, tilapia, or halibut)

Sea salt

Freshly ground black pepper

3 tablespoons butter, divided

1 large white onion, diced

2 large carrots, peeled and shredded

2 celery stalks, diced

1 green bell pepper, cored and diced

1 red bell pepper, cored and diced

3 garlic cloves, peeled and minced

1 (16-ounce) can crushed tomatoes, undrained

1 (16-ounce) bag fresh, baby spinach

1. Preheat the oven to 350°F.
2. Cut the fish into playing card–size pieces. Pat them dry, and season with salt and pepper.
3. In a large nonstick skillet over high heat, melt 1½ tablespoons of butter. Add the fish and cook for 1 minute on each side; it should be white and firm on the edges but not cooked through. Set aside on a plate.
4. In the same skillet over medium-high heat, melt the remaining 1½ tablespoons of butter and cook the onion, carrots, celery, bell peppers, and garlic until the onion is translucent, 3 to 5 minutes. Turn off the heat, and add the can of tomatoes and their juices. Mix well.
5. Cover the bottom of a small deep baking dish or Dutch oven with a layer of spinach, and arrange a layer of fish to cover the bottom of the dish. Top the fish with a layer of the vegetable mixture. Continue to layer with spinach and fish, finishing the top with the vegetable mixture.
6. Cover the baking dish with foil or an appropriate lid, bake for 45 minutes, until the fish is tender but flaky and the vegetable mixture is bubbling, and serve.

Storage Note: This dish keeps well and makes for tasty leftovers up to 3 days.

Recipe Tip: For an even richer dish, you can add ¼ cup of Homemade Almond Mayo (page 166) or plain Greek yogurt to the top before baking.

Per Serving Calories: 415; Total fat: 12g; Saturated fat: 6g; Sodium: 404mg; Carbohydrates: 29g; Fiber: 9g; Protein: 46g

Pesto Salmon, Green Beans, and Baby Reds

Serves 2 | Prep time: 20 minutes | Cook time: 40 minutes

This meal is a clean, healthy go-to; the pesto sauce brightens this dish and brings a lemony, nutty flavor to the tender pink salmon. The healthy fats in the fish and the easy-to-digest veggies make this recipe a gut-friendly winner.

FOR THE SALMON AND VEGGIES

5 or 6 small baby red potatoes, quartered

2 tablespoons coconut oil or ghee, melted, divided

Sea salt

Freshly ground black pepper

2 pieces wild-caught salmon (about playing card or palm size, about 1 pound total)

1 pound green beans, ends cut off, halved

FOR THE PESTO SAUCE

1 cup fresh basil leaves, loosely packed (about 1 to 2 handfuls)

3 garlic cloves, peeled

⅓ cup pine nuts

¼ cup olive oil

2 tablespoons freshly squeezed lemon juice

½ teaspoon sea salt

1. Preheat the oven to 325°F.
2. On a baking sheet, toss the baby red potatoes with 1 tablespoon of coconut oil, and liberally sprinkle with salt and pepper.
3. Roast in the oven for 35 to 40 minutes, or until tender and turning brown at the edges.
4. Meanwhile, make the pesto sauce. In a blender or food processor, combine the basil, garlic, pine nuts, olive oil, lemon juice, and salt, and blend until smooth.
5. Place the fish in a baking dish and sprinkle with salt and pepper. Using a spoon, scoop pesto atop each piece of fish; you'll use about 1 heaping tablespoon per piece.
6. Arrange the green beans around the fish. Drizzle the remaining tablespoon of coconut oil over the fish and green beans.
7. Bake for 15 to 20 minutes, or until the sides of the fish are no longer translucent pink.
8. Plate the fish and green beans together with a scoop of potatoes, and serve with a side of pesto for dipping.

Storage Note: The salmon and veggies keep, refrigerated and covered with a lid, for 4 to 5 days. You can also freeze this meal for easy lunches and dinners. Keep the pesto separate until ready to eat.

Recipe Tip: Try making pesto with arugula instead of basil for a different flavor.

Per Serving Calories: 899; Total fat: 63g; Saturated fat: 19g; Sodium: 605mg; Carbohydrates: 34g; Fiber: 11g; Protein: 56g

Lemon Butter Scallops over Wild Rice

Serves 2 | Prep time: 5 minutes | Cook time: 10 minutes | 5 Ingredients | NF | Quick Prep

You had me at lemon and butter! But wait; it gets better: The tender, melt-in-your-mouth scallops are succulent with a pop of garlic. The wild rice is saturated with the lemon butter sauce, and the whole thing is just a mouthful of joy. And the simplicity of this dish makes it very easy to digest. The scallops are packed with nutrients, and the healthy fat is just a bonus.

FOR THE SCALLOPS

1 pound sea scallops, fresh or
   frozen and thawed, rinsed

Sea salt

Freshly ground black pepper

1 tablespoon ghee

FOR THE LEMON BUTTER SAUCE

2 tablespoons ghee

3 garlic cloves, peeled
   and minced

1 teaspoon sea salt

1 teaspoon freshly ground
   black pepper

1 lemon, juiced

FOR SERVING

4 cups cooked wild rice

½ cup chopped fresh parsley

TO MAKE THE SCALLOPS

1. Pat the scallops dry, and sprinkle with salt and pepper.
2. In a large skillet over medium-high heat, melt the ghee. Add the scallops and cook for 1 to 2 minutes on each side, until they begin to brown on the edges and firm up. Set aside on a plate.

TO MAKE THE LEMON BUTTER SAUCE

In the same skillet, prepare the sauce. Melt the ghee, add the garlic, salt, and pepper, and sauté just until the garlic begins to brown. Add the lemon juice and deglaze the pan, scraping up any browned bits that may be on the bottom. Turn the heat off.

TO SERVE

1. Place 2 cups of wild rice in each bowl, top with a few cooked scallops, and drizzle with the lemon butter sauce.
2. Sprinkle with the chopped parsley and serve.

Storage Note: This dish will keep, refrigerated in an airtight container, for 2 to 3 days.

Recipe Tip: Add a few tablespoons of capers to the sauce for a tangy punch. These scallops are also delicious over a salad for lunch.

Per Serving Calories: 723; Total fat: 23g; Saturated fat: 12g; Sodium: 1,316mg; Carbohydrates: 81g; Fiber: 8g; Protein: 52g

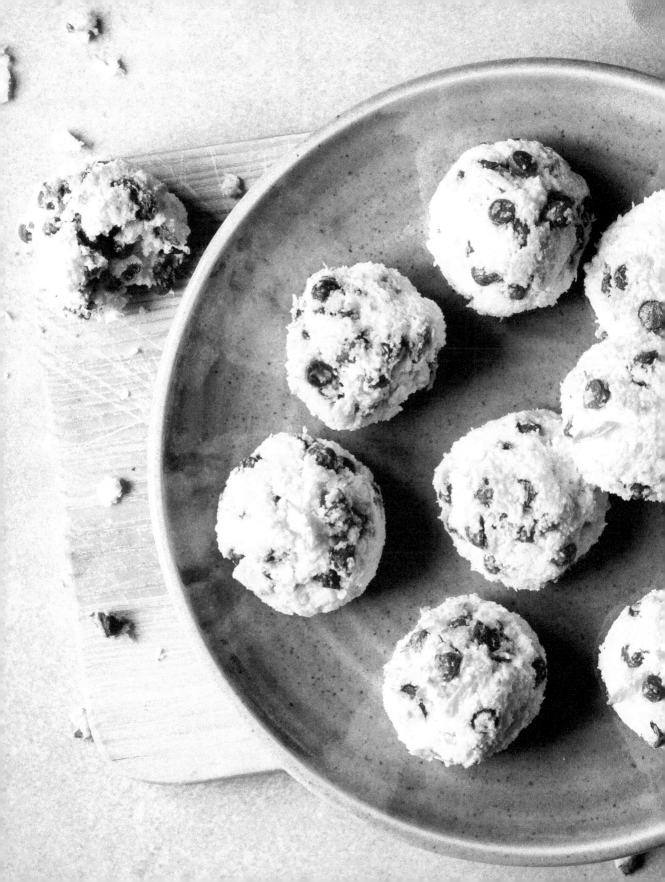

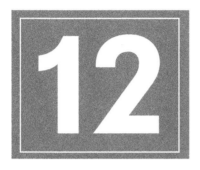

Dessert and Digestive Teas

Opposite: Almond-Coconut Haystacks, page 151

Green Apple Cashew Butter Bites

Serves 2 | Prep time: 10 minutes | 5 Ingredients | Paleo | Quick Prep | Vegan

Why green apples and not red? Green apples are lower in fructose, which can be less than friendly to the gut, and also contain a bit more fiber—which is what our friendly bacteria like to dine on. That makes this snack a winner with excellent crunchy/mushy and sweet/sour ratios.

1 large green apple
2 tablespoons cashew butter
¼ teaspoon ground cinnamon
¼ cup pomegranate seeds

1. Slice the apple horizontally into round slices, removing seeds and stem.
2. Use a butter knife to spread a thin layer of cashew butter onto each slice, like buttering toast.
3. Sprinkle each piece with some cinnamon, then top with pomegranate seeds.
4. Try stacking the slices back together to make 2 delicious towers and serve.

Storage Note: This snack will keep, refrigerated in an airtight container, for 4 to 5 days. This snack also travels well and doesn't have to be refrigerated throughout the day.

Recipe Tip: Not pomegranate season? Try using dried cranberries or goji berries instead.

Per Serving Calories: 162; Total fat: 8g; Saturated fat: 2g; Sodium: 4mg; Carbohydrates: 40g; Fiber: 4g; Protein: 3g

Almond-Coconut Haystacks

Makes 2 dozen small haystacks | Prep time: 35 minutes, plus 45 minutes to cool | Cook time: 50 minutes | 5 Ingredients | Paleo | Vegetarian

This Paleo-inspired dessert had me excited the moment I learned it involved coconut condensed milk. These treats are crumbly, sweet, crunchy, chewy, and basically perfect. Great for holidays and parties, they'll keep you honest with your diet. They aren't loaded with flour, sugar, or other typical dessert ingredients, so they don't inflame or irritate the gut. My kind of dessert!

FOR THE COCONUT CONDENSED MILK

1 (16-ounce) can full-fat coconut milk

4 tablespoons raw honey

Pinch sea salt (about ⅛ teaspoon)

FOR THE HAYSTACKS

½ cup sliced almonds

1 cup dark chocolate chips (sweetened with stevia; I like the brand Lily's)

1½ cups unsweetened shredded coconut

TO MAKE THE COCONUT CONDENSED MILK

1. Pour the coconut milk into a saucepan over medium-low heat. Add the honey and salt, and stir until melted.
2. Simmer the mixture for about 25 minutes, stirring occasionally as it begins to reduce and thicken. Turn off the heat and let it sit until totally cool.

TO MAKE THE ALMOND-COCONUT HAYSTACKS

1. Preheat the oven to 325°F.
2. In a large bowl, mix the almond slices, chocolate chips, shredded coconut, and coconut condensed milk.
3. Grease a mini muffin tin (ideal for keeping the haystacks together). If you don't have one, line a baking sheet with parchment paper.
4. Using wet fingers and a small spoon, drop a heaping teaspoon of the almond mixture into each muffin tin (or onto the cookie sheet), and repeat until you've used up all of the batter.
5. Bake for 20 to 25 minutes, or until the haystacks are golden brown and the chocolate chips look melted.
6. Completely cool and refrigerate before indulging, around 45 minutes. The wait will be worth it.

> **CONTINUED ON NEXT PAGE**

Almond-Coconut Haystacks

> **CONTINUED**

Storage Note: The haystacks will be firm and crumbly. Store them in an airtight container for up to a few weeks. They freeze well, too.

Recipe Tip: When the condensed milk begins to cool, moisture will gather on the surface. Tip the pan, and drain out the liquid. It helps the final haystacks stick together better in the oven. It is tempting to gorge on healthy treats when you are on a restrictive diet like this one. This recipe is meant as an indulgence; I recommend eating 3 small pieces when you make them and freezing the rest for later.

Per Serving (1 cookie) Calories: 133; Total fat: 11g; Saturated fat: 9g; Sodium: 13mg; Carbohydrates: 9g; Fiber: 2g; Protein: 2g

Cultured Blueberry-Coconut Pudding

Serves 4 | Prep time: 8 hours 30 minutes | 5 Ingredients | Paleo | Vegan

When you're first cleansing your gut, you may not be able to tolerate dairy very well. However, there's lots to love about the gut-friendly bacteria in cultured yogurt. This recipe gives you the best of both worlds, with lots of probiotics and easy-to-digest coconut milk.

4 cups coconut meat, cleaned of all the brown woody bits (from about 2 coconuts)

2 tablespoons coconut water kefir OR 1 packet kefir starter

¼ cup water

¼ teaspoon vanilla extract

1 tablespoon raw honey

1 cup fresh blueberries

1. In a blender, combine the coconut meat and coconut water kefir or starter. Blend until smooth and thick but not soupy. Add 1 tablespoon of water at a time to get a nice, smooth consistency.

2. Place the coconut mixture in a mixing bowl and cover with a cheesecloth or cotton kitchen towel. Keep at 72°F for 8 hours. If your house is cooler, you can place the bowl atop a heating pad on low.

3. After 8 hours, place the bowl in the fridge until chilled, at least 30 minutes.

4. Return the coconut mixture to the blender, and add the vanilla, honey, and blueberries. Blend until smooth.

5. Top with a few whole blueberries to serve.

Storage Note: This pudding will keep, refrigerated in an airtight container, for 4 to 5 days. While fermenting on your counter, it is important to keep the bowl covered and keep the mixture warm. If the temperature drops, the bacteria may go dormant and cease to ferment the coconut meat.

Recipe Tip: You may be relieved to find out that you can find frozen coconut meat online now. No more fussing with scooping the meat out of the coconuts yourself, although the process certainly makes the reward that much sweeter.

Per Serving Calories: 322; Total fat: 26g; Saturated fat: 24g; Sodium: 22mg; Carbohydrates: 22g; Fiber: 8g; Protein: 3g

Frozen Yogurt Blueberries

Makes 1 pint | Prep time: 10 minutes, plus 2 hours to freeze | 5 Ingredients | NF | Paleo | Vegetarian

This antioxidant-rich, guilt-free snack is fun to make and fun to eat—and your gut will be on board with how easy it is to digest.

1 cup plain Greek yogurt

1 tablespoon raw honey

1 pint blueberries, washed, drained, and patted dry with a paper towel

1. Line a baking sheet with parchment paper, and set out some wooden skewers or toothpicks.
2. In a small bowl, combine the yogurt and honey, and mix well.
3. Skewer the blueberries, and swirl them in the yogurt mixture until thickly coated.
4. Using a fork, push the blueberries off the skewer and onto the parchment.
5. Repeat until you have an army of yogurt-covered blueberries.
6. Place in the freezer for about 2 hours, or until frozen solid.
7. Eat as a snack, add to a salad, or use to top gluten-free oatmeal.

Storage Note: I keep these frozen in an airtight container so they stay firm. They will stay good for months and months!

Recipe Tip: You can try other flavors of yogurt if there is no sugar added. Greek yogurt is the best to use because of its thickness; other yogurts are too runny.

Per Serving (¼ cup) Calories: 57; Total fat: 1g; Saturated fat: 0g; Sodium: 13mg; Carbohydrates: 11g; Fiber: 1g; Protein: 3g

Cowboy Cookies

Makes 1 dozen cookies | Prep time: 5 minutes | Cook time: 15 minutes | Quick Prep | Vegan

I was introduced to cowboy cookies by an actual cowboy—well, a cowgirl. I was trail riding for a whole day, and guess what the snack was? After hours of riding in the heat, nothing was more delicious than this crunchy, sweet, chewy morsel. This is my healthy version, which is super gut-friendly and still delicious.

1½ cup gluten-free oats

½ teaspoon sea salt

2 teaspoons ground cinnamon

2 ripe bananas, mashed

1 teaspoon vanilla extract

⅓ cup chopped almonds

⅓ cup shredded coconut

⅓ cup stevia-sweetened chocolate chips

1. Preheat the oven to 350°F. Line a baking sheet with parchment paper.

2. In a medium mixing bowl, combine the oats, salt, and cinnamon. Add the bananas and vanilla, and mix well.

3. Stir in the almonds, coconut, and chocolate chips, and combine well.

4. Drop large scoops of the batter onto the parchment paper to make a dozen cookies; I use an ice cream scoop.

5. Bake for 12 to 15 minutes, or until golden brown. Cool before eating.

Storage Note: These cookies will keep in an airtight container for a week or in the freezer for a month.

Recipe Tip: It's tempting to overeat these. I suggest making mini-cookies so you can store lots of them in the freezer for later and take a few in a resealable plastic bag to work as a snack. I would limit your consumption during your diet to 4 full-size cookies per week.

Per Serving (1 cookie) Calories: 89; Total fat: 5g; Saturated fat: 2g; Sodium: 98mg; Carbohydrates: 13g; Fiber: 3g; Protein: 2g

Coffee-Coconut Creamsicles

Serves 4 | Prep time: 10 minutes, plus 2 hours to freeze | 5 Ingredients | Paleo | Vegan

Since you've given up coffee for this diet, I thought this healthy treat with a hint of coffee flavor might bring a little comfort to your palate. Coffee in tiny amounts can stimulate digestive function, and coupled with coconut fat, it becomes a powerful brain food. And, of course, feeding the brain always amounts to nourishing the gut.

4 dates, pitted

1 (16-ounce) can full-fat coconut milk

1 teaspoon instant coffee or coffee extract (I like to use 1 packet of Four Sigmatic Chaga mushroom "coffee")

½ teaspoon vanilla extract

1. Soak the dates in a cup of warm water for 5 minutes to soften.
2. In a blender, combine the soaked dates, coconut milk, coffee, and vanilla. Blend until smooth.
3. Pour into Popsicle molds, mini cupcake molds or freezer pop molds, and place in the freezer for about 2 hours, or until frozen.
4. Run warm water over the mold and remove to enjoy.

Storage Note: Keep frozen until ready to eat.

Recipe Tip: If you are sensitive to coffee, you can use raw cacao or stick to vanilla. Get creative with this recipe; it's such a fun treat, and you can stumble upon some gems. I once made a coconut, banana, and cinnamon blend that was also wonderful.

Per Serving Calories: 286; Total fat: 27g; Saturated fat: 24g; Sodium: 17mg; Carbohydrates: 12g; Fiber: 3g; Protein: 3g

Herbal Anti-Inflammatory Digestive Teas

Serves 2 | Prep time: 5 minutes | Cook time: 10 minutes | 5 Ingredients | DF | NF | Paleo | Quick Prep | Vegetarian

These 2 teas help reduce inflammation in the gut. They're best to have after a meal and again before bedtime. The turmeric and tart cherry have incredibly potent anti-inflammatory properties and can do wonders for all inflammatory gut issues. Tart cherry has even been known to resolve issues with gout.

TURMERIC TEA

4 cups water

1 teaspoon ground turmeric or 1 inch fresh turmeric, peeled and grated

1 pinch freshly ground black pepper

1 lemon wedge

TART CHERRY TEA

4 cups water

¼ cup organic tart cherry juice (not from concentrate; I use Smart Juice)

1 teaspoon raw honey

1 lemon wedge

TO MAKE THE TURMERIC TEA

1. In a medium saucepan, bring the water to a boil.
2. Add the turmeric, lower the heat, and simmer for 10 minutes.
3. Strain well.
4. Pour into 2 cups, add the pepper and a squeeze of lemon, and serve.

TO MAKE THE TART CHERRY TEA

1. In a medium saucepan, bring the water to a boil. Add the cherry juice and honey, and simmer for 5 minutes
2. Pour into 2 cups, and serve with a squeeze of lemon.

Storage Note: These teas are consumed immediately and drunk warm for maximum benefit and nutritional content. However, you can store the tea in an insulated container to keep it warm throughout the day, or even cool it and add to your water or drink as an iced tea.

Recipe Tip: These teas can be an acquired taste, so I'd like to remind you they are medicinal and not always meant to be enjoyed as a cup of hot chocolate might be. You will love the healing properties, which will bring you to love the flavor.

Per Serving Calories: 28; Total fat: 0g; Saturated fat: 0g; Sodium: 3mg; Carbohydrates: 7g; Fiber: 0g; Protein: 0g

Herbal Stimulating Digestive Teas

Serves 2 | Prep time: 5 minutes | Cook time: 10 minutes | 5 Ingredients | DF | NF | Paleo | Quick Prep | Vegetarian

These 2 teas help activate the digestive system by stimulating bile production and stomach juices and aiding in elimination. Ginger and peppermint are similar herbs that have soothing properties; peppermint can reduce gas and bloating almost instantly. Apple cider vinegar makes a microbe-loving, soothing tea that for centuries has been responsible for healing everything from gut ailments to arthritis.

GINGER-PEPPERMINT TEA

4 cups water

1 inch fresh ginger root, peeled and grated

½ cup fresh peppermint leaves

1 lemon wedge

APPLE CIDER VINEGAR TEA

2 cups sparkling mineral water (I like Gerolsteiner or Mountain Valley)

¼ cup raw, organic apple cider vinegar (I use Bragg's)

1 tablespoon raw honey

Juice of 2 limes

TO MAKE THE GINGER-PEPPERMINT TEA

1. In a medium saucepan, bring the water to a boil. Add the ginger, peppermint leaves, and lemon wedge. Reduce the heat to low, and simmer for 5 minutes. Remove from the heat, cover, and allow to steep for 5 more minutes.
2. Strain into 2 cups and sip.

TO MAKE THE APPLE CIDER VINEGAR TEA

1. In a medium saucepan over low heat, combine the mineral water, vinegar, honey and lime juice. Stir until the honey has melted, then take off heat. DO NOT BRING TO A BOIL.
2. Pour into 2 cups and sip slowly.
3. You can use regular water, but the sparkling water gives this tea a slightly soda-like flavor that makes it a bit of a treat.

Storage Note: These teas are consumed immediately and enjoyed warm for maximum benefit and nutritional content. However, you can store the tea in an insulated container to keep it warm throughout the day, or even cool it and add to your water or drink as an iced tea.

Recipe Tip: These teas can be an acquired taste, so I'd like to remind you they are medicinal and not always meant to be enjoyed as a cup of hot chocolate might be. You will love the healing properties, which will bring you to love the flavor.

Per Serving Calories: 50; Total fat: 0g; Saturated fat: 0g; Sodium: 1mg; Carbohydrates: 14g; Fiber: 0g; Protein: 0g

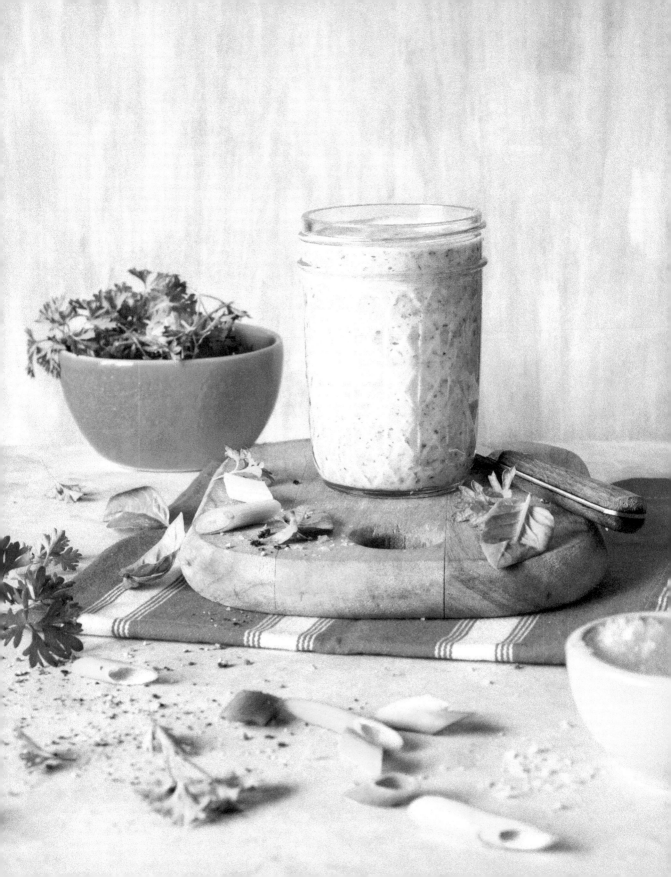

13

Basic Staples, Condiments, and Dressings

Opposite: Green Goddess Dressing, page 164

161

Seed Bread

Serves 4 | Prep time: 10 minutes, plus overnight to soak (optional) | Cook time: 1 hour | Paleo | Quick Prep | Vegetarian

I acquired this recipe from an Icelandic friend of mine. It is incredibly delicious, hearty, and extremely nutritious. The fiber and healthy fats in this bread will leave your microbes screaming for more.

½ cup almonds

½ cup walnuts

½ cup pumpkin seeds

½ cup sunflower seeds

½ cup sesame seeds

½ cup flaxseed

5 large eggs

½ cup coconut oil or ghee

2 teaspoons sea salt

1. Preheat the oven to 350°F.
2. In a large bowl, combine the almonds, walnuts, pumpkin seeds, sunflower seeds, sesame seeds, flaxseed, eggs, coconut oil, and salt. Mix well.
3. Line a bread pan with parchment paper. Pour the batter into the pan, and tap on the counter to distribute.
4. Bake for 1 hour, or until a toothpick inserted into the center comes out clean.
5. Slice and serve.

Storage Note: This bread will keep in an airtight container on the counter for a week or refrigerated for 2 weeks. You can also freeze it for up to 2 months.

Recipe Tip: Nuts are incredibly nutritious, but they can be tough for some people to digest. I recommend soaking the pumpkin and sunflower seeds, almonds, and walnuts overnight. Strain them and pat dry before using.

Per Serving Calories: 812; Total fat: 75g; Saturated fat: 30g; Sodium: 1,252mg; Carbohydrates: 20g; Fiber: 11g; Protein: 24g

5-Ingredient Flatbread

Serves 4 | Prep time: 5 minutes | Cook time: 10 minutes | 5 Ingredients | DF | Paleo | Quick Prep | Vegetarian

This recipe is easy to make and really takes care of that craving we all have for bread when trying to stick to a gluten-free lifestyle. You can also flavor it by mixing in garlic powder, rosemary, or other herbs and spices.

12 large egg whites

¼ cup coconut flour

2 teaspoons baking powder

1 teaspoon sea salt

1 teaspoon coconut
    oil, divided

1. In a large mixing bowl, whisk the egg whites for 1 minute, then add the coconut flour, baking powder, and salt. Make sure there are no lumps.

2. In a large skillet with a lid over medium-high heat, melt ¼ teaspoon of coconut oil.

3. Scoop about ½ cup of the egg mixture into the pan, and cover immediately.

4. Check frequently for bubbles beginning to form on the bread. When they do, after about 1 to 2 minutes, flip it over.

5. Repeat with the remaining coconut oil and batter until all batter has been used; you should have 3 or 4 flatbreads.

Storage Note: Best eaten immediately, but you can refrigerate for up to 1 week.

Recipe Tip: I eat these flatbreads with the Quinoa Kibbeh (page 132) and with the Kalua Pork (page 130). You can also cut them into small triangles and dip them into Cucumber Laban (page 171) as an appetizer, or heat them in the oven to serve with hummus.

Per Serving Calories: 124; Total fat: 3g; Saturated fat: 2g; Sodium: 683mg; Carbohydrates: 12g; Fiber: 6g; Protein: 13g

Green Goddess Dressing

Serves 4 | Prep time: 10 minutes | NF | Paleo | Quick Prep | Vegetarian

I always have this dressing handy. It's capable of turning anything bland into a gourmet meal. It is filled with healthy herbs and spices that are easy to digest; some even stimulate healthy digestion. And the stems of almost all herbs are filled with beneficial bacteria called *Plantarum*.

1 cup fresh basil leaves

1 cup fresh parsley

1 cup Greek yogurt

2 tablespoons chopped scallions, white and green parts

2 garlic cloves, peeled and minced

1 teaspoon sea salt

½ teaspoon apple cider vinegar (I use Bragg's)

½ teaspoon freshly ground black pepper

Juice of 1 lemon

2 tablespoons olive oil

1. In a blender, combine the basil, parsley, yogurt, scallions, garlic, salt, vinegar, pepper, and lemon juice. Blend on medium until smooth.
2. Slowly add the olive oil as the blender continues to spin. This helps the oil to incorporate well and not simply stay at the top.
3. Transfer to an airtight jar, or drizzle onto a salad.

Storage Note: This dressing will keep, refrigerated, in an airtight jar, for up to 1 month. You can also freeze it in small containers and have plenty for your entire 4-week diet.

Recipe Tip: This dressing can be used as a dipping sauce, a sandwich spread, or a marinade for chicken or meat. I drizzle it on vegetable bowls and tacos or over sweet potatoes. Make plenty!

Per Serving Calories: 113; Total fat: 8g; Saturated fat: 2g; Sodium: 505mg; Carbohydrates: 4g; Fiber: 1g; Protein: 7g

Creamy Lemon-Tahini Dressing

Serves 4 | Prep time: 5 minutes | 5 Ingredients | NF | Paleo | Quick Prep | Vegan

Here's another staple to help give a flavor boost to almost any food. This sauce is loaded with gut-friendly nutrients and bursting with lemony flavor.

2 tablespoons tahini paste (sesame seed butter)

2 garlic cloves, peeled

Juice of 1 lemon

¼ teaspoon sea salt

2 tablespoons olive oil

1. In a food processor or blender, combine the tahini, garlic, lemon juice, salt, and oil.
2. Blend until smooth, adding water as needed to get a pourable, dressing-like consistency.

Storage Note: Store in an airtight jar for up to 2 weeks.

Recipe Tip: I like to leave this dressing thick and only add water as I need it, depending on the recipe. I add more water for a salad dressing or to drizzle over some wild rice, and I leave it thick if I am going to marinate a piece of fish.

Per Serving Calories: 110; Total fat: 11g; Saturated fat: 2g; Sodium: 159mg; Carbohydrates: 2g; Fiber: 1g; Protein: 2g

Homemade Almond Mayo

Makes 2 cups | Prep time: 20 minutes, plus overnight to soak | 5 Ingredients | Paleo | Vegan

A healthier mayonnaise is better for your digestion, and you'll never know the difference. It's creamy and tangy and can be used in the same ways as regular mayo: on a sandwich, in a tuna salad, as a raw veggie dip at parties, with baby red potatoes, or in my favorite, Deviled Egg Salad (page 82).

½ cup raw almonds

¼ teaspoon garlic powder

¾ teaspoon sea salt

½ to ¾ cup water

1 cup flax oil

3 tablespoons freshly squeezed lemon juice

½ teaspoon unpasteurized apple cider vinegar

1. In a medium bowl, soak the almonds overnight.
2. In the morning, slip the skins off the almonds and pat the almonds with a paper towel until dry.
3. In a blender or food processor, pulse the almonds into a fine powder.
4. Add the garlic powder and salt, and blend well.
5. Add the water, and blend until creamy.
6. Keep your blender or processor on low, and very slowly drizzle in the oil until the mixture thickens.
7. Add the lemon juice and vinegar, and blend for 1 minute, or until the mixture has a mayonnaise consistency.

Storage Note: This recipe will keep refrigerated in an airtight container for 2 weeks.

Recipe Tip: If you have a tree nut allergy, replace the ½ cup of almonds with 2 egg yolks. Also, note that the slower you drizzle the oil into the mixture, the creamier the texture becomes.

Per Serving (1 tablespoon) Calories: 69; Total Fat: 8g; Saturated Fat: 1g; Sodium: 55mg; Carbohydrates: 0g; Fiber: 0g; Protein: 0g

Dill and Caraway Sauerkraut

Makes 2 quarts | Prep time: 30 minutes, plus 3 to 7 days to ferment | 5 Ingredients | NF | Paleo | Vegan

Some people are intimidated by fermented vegetables. It's time to get over that fear! They are a magical, curative, and incredibly affordable food to accompany you along your healing journey. A study revealed that one serving of fermented foods was equal in probiotic content to an entire bottle of high-quality probiotic supplements. You can start with this very easy recipe.

1 bunch fresh dill

3½ cups water

1 tablespoon sea salt

1 culture starter (I use Body Ecology) (optional, see tip; omit for DF/Vegan or use a vegan starter)

2 green cabbages, cored and shredded with a food processor or using a knife

1 teaspoon caraway seeds

1. In a blender, combine the dill, water, salt, and starter (if using). Blend until liquefied.

2. In a large mixing bowl, combine the shredded cabbage, caraway seeds, and dill mixture.

3. Squeeze and massage the cabbage thoroughly until additional liquid collects in the bowl and the cabbage is not as firm.

4. Pack tightly into 1-quart mason jars. Cap each loosely with a lid—don't fully tighten.

5. Store in a large plastic container to catch any leaks from the jars, which are not uncommon.

6. Store at 72°F for 3 to 7 days (see recipe tip). The longer you leave the sauerkraut, the more potent in probiotic content it will become. Taste at intervals during the last few days, and when you like the flavor, screw the caps down tightly and refrigerate before enjoying.

Storage Note: This will keep, refrigerated and unopened, for a few months. Once opened, the sauerkraut can stay refrigerated for up to 1 month.

> **CONTINUED ON NEXT PAGE**

Dill and Caraway Sauerkraut

> **CONTINUED**

Recipe Tip: I use a heating pad under the jars to maintain 72°F or warmer; otherwise, the bacteria may go dormant and stop fermenting the vegetables. Expect some leaking, but do NOT tighten the jar lids too tightly or they may crack. If you have a gut-related disorder, it is best to start with 1 tablespoon of fermented vegetables and work your way up each week. You can expect some tolerable bloating that should subside the more you consume them. Vegetables will ferment with sea salt only; the culture starter is optional. However, when healing the gut, it is wise to add as many as possible of the specific strains of bacteria needed to help the healing process. Using a starter like Body Ecology Culture is a great idea.

Per Serving (1 cup) Calories: 7; Total fat: 0g; Saturated fat: 0g; Sodium: 707mg; Carbohydrates: 1g; Fiber: 1g; Protein: 0g

Dairy Kefir

Serves 4 | Prep time: 20 minutes, plus 18 to 24 hours to ferment | 5 Ingredients | NF | Vegetarian

You can't have a diet specific to healing the gut without fermented foods. Kefir is one of the most powerful, healing, and yummy fermented foods; people have been enjoying it for centuries. It is like a watery yogurt: sour, tangy, and a bit fizzy. You can acquire kefir grains if you choose, but these days you can also find starter products like Yogourmet. My favorite is the Body Ecology kefir starter, which can be purchased online. These bacteria are selected to specifically aid in gut health. I recommend enjoying half a cup of kefir before bed.

4 cups organic milk
(cow or goat)

½ cup heavy (whipping)
cream (optional, but makes
for a very creamy kefir)

1 packet kefir starter

1. In a medium saucepan, heat the milk and cream (if using) to 92°F. Be careful not to overheat; if you don't have a thermometer, you can use your finger to check the temperature. It should feel neutral to the touch, not hot or cold.
2. Pour the warm milk mixture into a blender. Add the kefir starter pack, and blend for a few seconds to mix the milk and starter.
3. Pour the liquid into a glass jar, and top with a tight-fitting lid.
4. Store at room temperature to ferment, ideally 72°F to 75°F, for 18 to 24 hours. It will thicken until slightly clumpy and have a distinctly sour aroma.
5. Refrigerate.

Storage Note: This drink can be refrigerated in a sealed container for up to 2 weeks.

Recipe Tip: Using the kefir in a smoothie, in a dressing, or as a quick snack is a great way to boost nutrition in your meals. If you are a vegan or sensitive to dairy, check out the Fermented Coconut Water Kefir recipe on page 170.

Per Serving Calories: 148; Total fat: 8g; Saturated fat: 5g; Sodium: 103mg; Carbohydrates: 11g; Fiber: 0g; Protein: 8g

Fermented Coconut Water Kefir

Serves 4 | Prep time: 20 minutes, plus 1 to 3 days to ferment | 5 Ingredients | Paleo | Vegan

Although dairy foods like kefir or yogurt are an excellent way to get massive doses of healthy probiotics, not all of us tolerate dairy well. If you're lactose intolerant, or simply want to cut down on dairy, try this tasty fermented coconut drink instead.

4 to 6 cups coconut water (from young Thai coconuts or cartons of unpasteurized coconut water)

1 packet kefir starter (I use Body Ecology kefir starter)

1. In a medium saucepan over very low heat, heat the coconut water to 92°F. If you don't have a thermometer, you can use your finger to check the temperature. It should feel neutral to the touch, not hot or cold.
2. Pour the warm coconut water into a blender. Add the kefir starter packet. Blend quickly for a few seconds, then pour into a glass container with a tight-fitting lid.
3. Store at 72°F or warmer for 1 to 3 days.
4. Chill and drink. If you are new to kefir, start with 2 ounces daily and work your way up to 6 ounces per day.

Storage Note: This will keep, refrigerated in an airtight container, for up to 2 weeks.

Recipe Tip: You can use ¼ cup of your first batch as a starter to begin another batch and can do this up to 7 times before it starts to lose potency. This goes for dairy kefir, as well.

Per Serving Calories: 75; Total fat: 1g; Saturated fat: 1g; Sodium: 383mg; Carbohydrates: 15g; Fiber: 4g; Protein: 3g

Cucumber Laban

Serves 1 | Prep time: 10 minutes | 5 Ingredients | NF | Paleo | Quick Prep | Vegetarian

This Middle Eastern sauce is one of my favorite refreshing sides. It brightens everything you dip in it with a lemony, minty tang. And let's not forget about all the gut-loving microbes that come in Greek yogurt! This pairs well with lamb, veggies, and fish.

2 cups plain Greek yogurt

3 Persian cucumbers, minced

Juice of 1 lemon

2 tablespoons fresh mint leaves, minced

2 garlic cloves, peeled and minced

½ teaspoon sea salt

¼ teaspoon freshly ground black pepper

In a small bowl, combine the yogurt, cucumbers, lemon, mint, garlic, salt, and pepper. Mix well.

Storage Note: This will keep, refrigerated in an airtight container, for up to 2 weeks.

Recipe Tip: I find the texture of this sauce is best when everything is finely minced or shredded.

Per Serving Calories: 442; Total fat: 7g; Saturated fat: 4g; Sodium: 1,154mg; Carbohydrates: 49g; Fiber: 6g; Protein: 51g

Gomashio (Japanese Sesame Seed Salt with Seaweed Topping)

Makes 2 cups | Prep time: 5 minutes | Cook time: 5 minutes | 5 Ingredients | NF | Paleo | Quick Prep | Vegan

Sesame seeds are tiny seeds packed with big nutrition that can support everything from blood pressure to bone health and hormones. Sesame has loads of fiber, so our guts love these little guys, and so should you. Add some mineral-rich kelp and sea salt, and you've got a wonderful topping for almost any dish.

1 cup sesame seeds

2 teaspoons sea salt

1 cup dried kelp flakes

1. In a large dry skillet over medium-high heat, toss the sesame seeds, salt, and kelp flakes, toasting until the mixture becomes fragrant, 2 to 3 minutes.
2. Transfer the mixture to a blender, and blend well.
3. Transfer to an airtight jar.

Storage Note: Store in your pantry for up to 3 weeks. Keep away from light as much as possible.

Recipe Tip: I save an old spice jar with a sprinkle top and use it to store my Gomashio. Sprinkle this mixture on everything from yogurt to salads, soups to desserts, and even oatmeal.

Per Serving (2 teaspoons) Calories: 18; Total fat: 2g; Saturated fat: 0g; Sodium: 85mg; Carbohydrates: 1g; Fiber: 0g; Protein: 1g

Fermented Salsa

Serves 4 | Prep time: 20 minutes, plus 48 hours to ferment | NF | Paleo | Vegan

You may have wondered by now why I don't include many tomatoes in this diet; they are quite acidic and can trigger inflammation in the stomach. They are also from the nightshade family, which tends to be inflammatory. However, when they are fermented, they become more nutritious and their inflammatory properties are neutralized by the lacto-fermentation process. Once fermented, tomatoes become healing to the gut, as do the peppers. So enjoy this gut-loving salsa.

2 pounds tomatoes, preferably Roma, though any will do

1 packet culture starter (optional; I like Body Ecology)

1 large onion

2 serrano peppers, seeded, membranes removed

1 jalapeño pepper, seeded, membranes removed

4 garlic cloves, peeled

1 bunch fresh cilantro

Juice of 2 limes

1 tablespoon sea salt

1. In a food processor or blender, combine the tomatoes, starter, onion, peppers, garlic, cilantro, lime juice, and salt. Pulse until chunky and a bit watery, but well combined.

2. Transfer to an airtight jar for 48 hours at room temperature, about 72°F.

3. Refrigerate.

Storage Note: This salsa will keep, refrigerated, in an airtight jar for up to 2 weeks.

Recipe Tip: These chile peppers can be very spicy, and it's hard to tell which are the hot ones. If you are very sensitive to hot chile peppers, I recommend using bell peppers of different colors. It's just as delicious.

Per Serving Calories: 73; Total fat: 1g; Saturated fat: 0g; Sodium: 1,419mg; Carbohydrates: 17g; Fiber: 5g; Protein: 3g

The Dirty Dozen and the Clean Fifteen™

A nonprofit environmental watchdog organization called Environmental Working Group (EWG) looks at data supplied by the US Department of Agriculture (USDA) and the Food and Drug Administration (FDA) about pesticide residues. Each year it compiles a list of the best and worst pesticide loads found in commercial crops. You can use these lists to decide which fruits and vegetables to buy organic to minimize your exposure to pesticides and which produce is considered safe enough to buy conventionally. This does not mean they are pesticide-free, though, so wash these fruits and vegetables thoroughly. The list is updated annually, and you can find it online at EWG.org/FoodNews.

Dirty Dozen™

1. strawberries
2. spinach
3. kale
4. nectarines
5. apples
6. grapes
7. peaches
8. cherries
9. pears
10. tomatoes
11. celery
12. potatoes

†Additionally, nearly three-quarters of hot pepper samples contained pesticide residues.

Clean Fifteen™

1. avocados
2. sweet corn
3. pineapples
4. sweet peas (frozen)
5. onions
6. papayas
7. eggplants
8. asparagus
9. kiwis
10. cabbages
11. cauliflower
12. cantaloupes
13. broccoli
14. mushrooms
15. honeydew melons

Conversion Tables

Volume Equivalents (Liquid)

Standard	US Standard (ounces)	Metric (approximate)
2 tablespoons	1 fl. oz.	30 mL
¼ cup	2 fl. oz.	60 mL
½ cup	4 fl. oz.	120 mL
1 cup	8 fl. oz.	240 mL
1½ cups	12 fl. oz.	355 mL
2 cups or 1 pint	16 fl. oz.	475 mL
4 cups or 1 quart	32 fl. oz.	1 L
1 gallon	128 fl. oz.	4 L

Volume Equivalents (Dry)

Standard	Metric (approximate)
⅛ teaspoon	0.5 mL
¼ teaspoon	1 mL
½ teaspoon	2 mL
¾ teaspoon	4 mL
1 teaspoon	5 mL
1 tablespoon	15 mL
¼ cup	59 mL
⅓ cup	79 mL
½ cup	118 mL
⅔ cup	156 mL
¾ cup	177 mL
1 cup	235 mL
2 cups or 1 pint	475 mL
3 cups	700 mL
4 cups or 1 quart	1 L

Oven Temperatures

Fahrenheit (F)	Celsius (C) (approximate)
250°	120°
300°	150°
325°	165°
350°	180°
375°	190°
400°	200°
425°	220°
450°	230°

Weight Equivalents

Standard	Metric (approximate)
½ ounce	15 g
1 ounce	30 g
2 ounces	60 g
4 ounces	115 g
8 ounces	225 g
12 ounces	340 g
16 ounces or 1 pound	455 g

Resources

"Stuff Your Doctor Should Know" podcast, hosted by author Kitty Martone: a diverse and varied array of nutritional information, world-renowned authors, scientists, and regular people with incredible journeys

For high-quality nutraceutical supplement recommendations without any toxic preservatives or excipients, go to http://www.healthygutgirl.com and click on the "shop" page.

Autism Recovery & BEDROK community: For more information on recovery of autism in children through diet, join the BEDROK community. http://www.bedrokcommunity.org

Download the low FODMAP diet app for IBS support, with the largest FODMAP food database available: https://www.monashfodmap.com/i-have-ibs/get-the-app

Weston Price Foundation: An excellent source for accurate information on nutrition and health, always aiming to provide the scientific validation of traditional food. http://westonaprice.org

"The Bright Side" with Ben Fuchs: The Bright Side with Pharmacist Ben is a fast-paced, entertaining, and educational radio program that focuses on the latest cutting-edge ideas in health and fitness, guaranteed to be a fun hour of weekly radio that will improve lives and empower day-to-day living: http://pharmacistben.com/bright-side-radio

BOOKS

The Body Ecology Diet
Donna Gates, MEd, ABAAHP, is the international best-selling author of this book, which is subtitled *Recovering Your Health and Rebuilding Your Immunity*. An advanced fellow with the American Academy of Anti-Aging Medicine, she is on a mission to change the way the world eats.

Gut and Psychology Syndrome
Dr. Natasha Campbell-McBride holds a degree in medicine and postgraduate degrees in nutrition. In her clinic in Cambridge, she specializes in nutrition for children and adults with behavioral issues and learning disabilities, and for adults with digestive and immune system disorders.

Nourishing Traditions
Author Sally Fallon, founder of the Weston Price Foundation, filled this book with old-school recipes and encourages us to look to our ancestors' recipes and ways for healing and balance.

References

Anxiety and Depression Association of America (ADAA). "Facts & Statistics." Accessed April 3, 2019. https://adaa.org/about-adaa/press-room/facts-statistics.

Bastyr Center for Natural Health. "Underlying Cause for Many Digestive Issues Is SIBO." February 16, 2016. https://bastyrcenter.org/about/news/2016/02/underlying-cause-many-digestive-issues-sibo.

Case-Lo, Christine, and Brian Wu. "Sensitivity Analysis: Purpose, Procedure, and Results." February 24, 2016. https://www.healthline.com/health/sensitivity-analysis#results.

Fox News. "Survey Shows 74 Percent of Americans Living with GI Discomfort." November 24, 2013. Last modified October 28, 2015. https://www.foxnews.com/health/survey-shows-74-percent-of-americans-living-with-gi-discomfort.

Gibson, P. R., and S. J. Shepherd. "Personal View: Food for Thought—Western Lifestyle and Susceptibility to Crohn's Disease. The FODMAP Hypothesis." *Alimentary Pharmacology and Therapeutics* 21, no. 12 (2005): 1399–1409. doi:10.1111/j.1365-2036.2005.02506.x.

Gogineni, Vijaya K., Lee E. Morrow, Philip J. Gregory, and Mark A. Malasker. "Probiotics: History and Evolution." *Journal of Ancient Diseases & Preventive Remedies* 1, no. 02 (2013). doi:10.4172/2329-8731.1000107. Available from: https://www.longdom.org/open-access/probiotics-history-and-evolution-2329-8731.1000107.pdf

Harvard Health. "Can Gut Bacteria Improve Your Health?" Last modified October 2016. https://www.health.harvard.edu/staying-healthy/can-gut-bacteria-improve-your-health

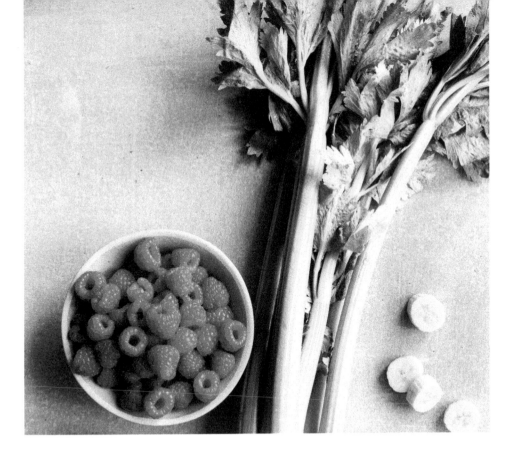

Johns Hopkins University. "Irritable Bowel Syndrome (IBS): Introduction." 2013. Available from: https://www.hopkinsmedicine.org/gastroenterology _hepatology/_pdfs/small_large_intestine/irritable_bowel_byndrome_IBS.pdf

Johns Hopkins University. "The Brain-Gut Connection." Accessed April 3, 2019. https://www.hopkinsmedicine.org/health/healthy_aging/healthy_body /the-brain-gut-connection.

National Institutes of Health (NIH). "NIH Human Microbiome Project Defines Normal Bacterial Makeup of the Body." June 13, 2012. https://www .nih.gov/news-events/news-releases/nih-human-microbiome-project -defines-normal-bacterial-makeup-body.

Salleh, Mohd Razali. "Life Event, Stress, and Illness." *The Malaysian Journal of Medical Sciences* 15, no. 4 (2008): 9–18. Available from: https://www.ncbi.nlm.nih .gov/pmc/articles/PMC3341916

Index

Acknowledgments

I would like to acknowledge the parents, both at the center I mentioned in the introduction but also my clients over the years, parents with children who suffer with digestive disorders and imbalances, including my own. My mother was one of these superheroes who was raising two other children who were older and healthy, and along comes Kitty, the runt. Ongoing chronic illness, sleepless nights, visits to the hospital, administering medications at all hours of the night and countless trips to the ER, always trying to find natural remedies and ways to ease my suffering. Mom, you are my hero, and without those tough years as a child and without the experiences I had with the children at the center and their parents, I would not be who I am today. Those were valuable experiences beyond anything I can express here. If you can tackle those issues with your children and raise a family and have a job and still put dinner on the table, the least I can do is teach people what I have learned. Thank you.

About the Author

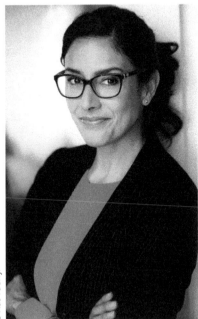

© Kat Tuohy.

KITTY MARTONE is a holistic health practitioner, a master herbalist, and a chef. With this background, and using her own health challenges as stepping stones to further her education, she has learned and will continue to learn about the ever-changing world of the human microbiome and how it is the conductor of our health and wellness. During her darkest days with her own health challenges, she prayed for guidance—the kind of guidance that she now offers through her podcast, *Stuff Your Doctor Should Know*, and through her thriving healing practice and writing. It is a dream come true for her to be able to connect you with alternative methods of healing, scientists on the cutting edge of their field of work, and so much more.

You can join the Healthy Gut Girl community here:
Website: www.healthygutgirl.com
Facebook: Healthy Gut Girl
Facebook: Estrogen Dominance Support Group
iTunes: Stuff Your Doctor Should Know
Instagram: @healthygutgirl_